MRCOG Part 1 Success Manual

I would like to dedicate this book to my beloved mother, who taught me the meaning and joy of giving to others, a concept so integral to teaching.

Khaldoun Sharif

Commissioning Editor: Ellen Green/Pauline Graham
Development Editor: Hannah Kenner
Project Manager: Jess Thompson
Design Direction: Louis Forgione
Illustration Manager: Bruce Hogarth

MRCOG Part 1
Success Manual

Khaldoun W. Sharif
MBBCh(Hons) MD FRCOG MFFP
Consultant Obstetrician and Gynaecologist
Clinical Director of Gynaecology and Assisted Conception Unit
RCOG Tutor
Birmingham Women's Hospital;
Honorary Senior Lecturer in Obstetrics and Gynaecology
University of Birmingham

Harry Gee
MD FRCOG
Consultant Obstetrician
Medical Director
Birmingham Women's Hospital

Martin J. Whittle
MD FRCOG FRCP
Professor of Fetal Medicine
Head of Division of Reproductive and Child Health
Associate Dean (Education)
University of Birmingham

Edinburgh   London   New York   Oxford   Philadelphia   St Louis   Sydney   Toronto   2008

SAUNDERS
ELSEVIER

An imprint of Elsevier Limited
©2008, Elsevier Limited. All rights reserved.

First published 2008

ISBN-13: 978-0-7020-2883-0

Some of the material in this book was previously published as:
Sharif K., Gee H. & Whittle M. MRCOG: Part 1 MCQs - Basic Science for Obstetrics and Gynaecology ISBN 0-7020-1970-4
Sharif K. MRCOG Survival Guide ISBN 0-7020-2545-3

British Library Cataloguing in Publication Data

A catalogue record for this book is available from the British Library

Library of Congress Cataloging in Publication Data

A catalog record for this book is available from the Library of Congress

Note

Knowledge and best practice in this field are constantly changing. As new research and experience broaden our knowledge, changes in practice, treatment and drug therapy may become necessary or appropriate. Readers are advised to check the most current information provided (i) on procedures featured or (ii) by the manufacturer of each product to be administered, to verify the recommended dose or formula, the method and duration of administration, and contraindications. It is the responsibility of the practitioner, relying on their own experience and knowledge of the patient, to make diagnoses, to determine dosages and the best treatment for each individual patient, and to take all appropriate safety precautions. To the fullest extent of the law, neither the Publisher nor the Authors assume any liability for any injury and/or damage to persons or property arising out of or related to any use of the material contained in this book.

The Publisher

Working together to grow
libraries in developing countries

www.elsevier.com | www.bookaid.org | www.sabre.org

ELSEVIER   BOOK AID International   Sabre Foundation

your source for books, journals and multimedia in the health sciences

www.elsevierhealth.com

Printed in China

Contents

Preface

Knowledge of basic sciences is a necessary foundation for the sound clinician. How else would you know where exactly to place your scalpel if you do not know the anatomy, and how could you prescribe drugs safely if you are not conversant with their pharmacokinetics and pharmacodynamics? Almost all postgraduate medical degrees have a basic science component in their assessment. The Royal College of Obstetricians and Gynaecologists in London tests its Membership (MRCOG) candidates in basic sciences during the Part 1 examination. However, the fact that this basic science knowledge is necessary does not mean it is easily acquired. Only one in three candidates pass the Part 1 MRCOG exam. Hence there is a need for detailed guidance on how to prepare for the exam and succeed: a Success Manual.

This manual is written primarily for the Part 1 MRCOG candidates. It should also be of help to candidates sitting other preliminary examinations in specialist obstetrics and gynaecology, such as the Membership of the Royal Australian College of Obstetricians and Gynaecologists, and the Arab Board Examination in Obstetrics and Gynaecology.

In writing this manual we have focused on two main goals. First and foremost, we realize that the most important aim is to pass the Part 1 MRCOG examination. Hence all the questions contained here are of similar content and format to those that you could be asked in the examination. Second, we believe that the retention of facts will increase significantly if the bases for them are clearly understood. Therefore, many of the provided answers attempt to explain the practical application of the facts as they relate to the field of clinical obstetrics and gynaecology.

Although the short-term objective is to pass the Part 1 exam, one should not lose sight of the longer-term aim, which is to become a better doctor, more capable of serving the patient. To that, we should all strive.

KWS, HG, MJW. 2007

How to use this book

In order to pass the Part 1 MRCOG exam (or any other exam, for that matter) you need to follow a number of steps:

- understand the exam system, regulations, and syllabus
- understand how to deal with the questions
- practise questions on each part of the syllabus, find out what is the right answer and why it is the right answer
- and then do more practice.

This book provides you with all those steps. Chapters 1–3 explain the examination regulations, system, syllabus and how to prepare. Chapter 4 takes you through MCQ techniques. Chapters 5–13 provide you with Part 1 exam-like questions on all branches of basic sciences relevant to obstetrics and gynaecology, together with their detailed explanatory answers. Chapter 14 has three full exam-like papers to do more practice, with the answers provided to mark your performance. Hopefully, all this will help you pass the Part 1 exam, and Chapter 15 advises you on what do after that.

1

Regulations

Introduction

It is generally accepted that knowledge of basic science is a prerequisite to sound clinical practice. The Royal College of Obstetricians and Gynaecologists (RCOG), in line with other Royal Colleges, tests its Membership candidates in basic science subjects related to the speciality. Previously, the MRCOG examination consisted of one part. However, since 1970 the examination has been divided into two parts: a basic science Part 1 and a clinically oriented Part 2. Although several changes have occurred in the format of Part 1 over the past three decades, the concept of a basic science examination is here to stay. The average overall pass rate in the Part 1 examination is around 35%. In this chapter we will explain and discuss the regulations for the Part 1 MRCOG examination. However, you should be aware that these are subject to regular review and you should check the College website (*http://www.rcog.org.uk*) for the latest regulations. Another useful source of recent changes is the MRCOG Blog on *http://web.mac.com/k.sharif*. This is a blogging site that discusses recent MRCOG regulations, hot topics, debatable issues and difficult and common questions.

Eligibility

Candidates are eligible to enter for the Part 1 examination when they have obtained their medical degree. The previous requirement of being registered as a medical practitioner was abolished by the Council of the RCOG in June 1991. In practice, this means that you can sit the examination during your pre-registration training (before 1991 only post-registration doctors could apply). This has a very important implication for candidates. It is well recognized, from analysis of previous Part 1 examination results, that one of the most important factors that deter-mine how well candidates do in the examination is the interval between graduation and sitting the examination; the shorter the interval, the higher the chances of success. By abolishing the registration require-ment the RCOG has effectively allowed candidates to sit the Part 1 examination 1 year earlier than previously permitted, thus increasing the chances of success (at least theoretically). The message is clear: start preparing for the Part 1 as soon as possible after graduation.

Overseas Candidates

Most overseas candidates pass the Part 1 MRCOG examination at home before they come to the UK, and there are many good reasons for doing this. First, your chances of getting a job in the UK are significantly increased if you already have the Part 1. Second, you can never really concentrate on Part 2 preparation with the Part 1 examination hanging over your head. Third, the time you will spend in the UK is usually lim-ited and should not be 'wasted' trying to get the Part 1. Rather, having got the Part 1 at home, you should spend this time acquiring experience on Part 2 MRCOG and beyond.

Dates, Closing Dates and Centres

The Part 1 examination is held twice every year on the first Mondays of March and September. The closing dates for receiving the completed application forms are the preceding 1st December for the March exami-nation and the preceding 1st June for the September examination. *Late entries are not accepted.*

The examination is held at centres both in the United Kingdom (UK) and overseas. The UK centres always include London and a com-bination of other major cities such as Manchester, Glasgow, Belfast and Edinburgh. Overseas centres are more variable and in the past have included Ireland, Egypt, Hong Kong, India, Jordan, Kuwait, Malaysia, Nepal, Saudi Arabia, United Arab Emirates and the West Indies.

Entry Requirements and Application

Once you have decided that you want to apply for the Part 1, the next step is to write to the Examination Secretary at the RCOG (27 Sussex

Place, Regent's Park, London NW1 4RG, UK). The Examination Department will send you the following:

1. The membership regulation booklet. This contains the application forms, detailed instructions and up-to-date regulations.
2. A list of the dates, centres and fees for your intended examination. The fees are subject to annual review. The 2007 fees are £250 for UK and overseas centres.

The completed application form, together with the following documents, should be returned to the Examination Department no later than the closing date:

1. The original of the Medical Degree or an attested copy. The College will accept copies of certificates attested by the British Embassy, British High Commission, British Consulate, British Council, the university issuing the medical degree certificate or the candidate's own Embassy. If your original certificate is in a language other than English, an attested translated copy should be sent. To avoid confusion candidates must use the *same* surname (preferred or family name) and other names, as shown on their medical degree, in all correspondence with the Examination Department. Candidates wishing to enter under a name other than that shown on the medical degree must also provide their certificate of registration showing the name by which they wish to be registered as a candidate. Candidates who subsequently change their name for whatever reason must immediately inform the College with documentary evidence. A marriage certificate alone is not accepted as evidence of change of name as a medical practitioner.
2. The fees in Sterling (cheque or postal order).

Applications for entry to the examinations held in the British Isles must be made to the Examination Secretary of the College in London. Applications for entry to the examinations held outside the British Isles can be made either to the local organizer or to the Examination Secretary of the College in London.

After a few weeks you will receive an acknowledgement of your application and a personal registration number. This number MUST be quoted in any future correspondence with the College.

You must take evidence of identification, which should include your name and photograph (e.g. passport), to all sections of the Part 1 and Part 2 Membership examinations for scrutiny by the invigilators and examiners. Candidates who fail to produce satisfactory identification at the entry to an examination may not be allowed into that examination.

If you withdraw your application for a particular Part 1 examination after the closing date or do not appear you will forfeit the examination fee. Attendance at any part of an examination will count as an attempt.

Two to four weeks before the date of your examination you will receive full details about the examination venue and time, and how to fill the answer sheet.

Pass Rates and Number of Attempts

Currently there is no limit to the number of attempts allowed at the Part 1 examination. When the examination was first introduced in 1970, the number of attempts was also unlimited. However, analysis of the results of the first few examinations showed that the pass rate declined with an increased number of attempts. Candidates sitting the Part 1 examination for the first time had a pass rate of 55%, while those sitting their seventh attempt or over had a pass rate of less than 5%. Therefore, the allowed number of attempts was reduced to six in 1979 and further down to five in 1981.

In the early 1990s, analysis of the examination results showed that the pass rate remained fairly constant for all the attempts (Figure 1). Consequently, the Council of the RCOG decided in 1992 to amend the regulations again and allow an unlimited number of attempts.

Exemption from the Part 1 Examination

Historically, the College has allowed candidates who have passed certain local examinations in obstetrics and gynaecology to sit the Part 2 MRCOG examination without having passed Part 1 (provided that they have not attempted Part 1 and failed it).

The College has decided to end exemption status for those local examination boards from 1 January 2007. Candidates who pass the local examination after that date will still have to pass Part 1 in order

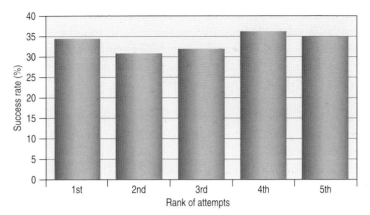

Figure 1 Pass rate in Part 1 versus rank of attempt

to sit the Part 2 MRCOG examination. Those candidates who have already passed their local examination by 1st January 2007 will have the usual ten-year period within which to sit Part 2 for the first time.

The reasons for discontinuing exemption are educational. The College has recently undertaken a review of its Part 1 MRCOG examination, which will result in changes in both the format and the content of the examination. The Part 1 and Part 2 MRCOG will form a single integrated blueprint derived from the new Curriculum for Core Training. It is therefore becoming increasingly difficult for overseas examinations to retain their comparability with an examination that is undergoing fundamental and rapid change.

The exempted local exams, and the dates from when the exemption began, are:

1. Part 1 examination (Obstetrics and Gynaecology), Arab Board for Medical Specializations, July 1996.

2. Primary examination for the Fellowship of the College of Obstetricians and Gynaecologists of South Africa (College of Medicine of South Africa), July 1972.

3. Primary examination, Fellowship of the Medical Council Obstetrics and Gynaecology (Nigeria Medical Council), February 1974.

4. Part 1 MS (Obstetrics and Gynaecology) examination, Post-graduate Institute of Medicine, University of Colombo, Sri Lanka, September 1983.

5. Part 1 examination (Obstetrics and Gynaecology), Fellowship of the College of Physicians and Surgeons of Pakistan, February 1985.

6. Primary examination (Obstetrics and Gynaecology), Fellowship of the West African College of Surgeons, July 1986.

7. Part 1 Clinical MD Sudan (Obstetrics and Gynaecology) examination, Sudan Medical Specialisation Board, October 2002 (or its predecessor, Part 1 Clinical MD (Obstetrics and Gynaecology) examination, University of Khartoum, January 1989).

8. Part 1 MD examination, Al Arab Medical University, Libya, September 1988.

9. Part 1 Master of Obstetrics and Gynaecology examination (UKM/UM), Malaysia, September 1996.

10. Part 1 examination for the Fellowship of the Bangladesh College of Physicians and Surgeons, May 1999.

11. Fellowship of the Iraqi Board of Obstetrics and Gynaecologists (FIBOG) – Part 1, December 2004.

12. First Year Master of Medical Science (Obstetrics and Gynaecology) Examination – Basic Sciences for University of Medicine 1, 2, Mandalay and Defence Services Medical Academy, Myanmar, December 2004.

If you wish to apply for exemption from the Part 1 Membership examination you should submit the original letter (or attested copy) confirming success in one of the above examinations, medical degree certificate and certificate of registration as a medical practitioner (originals or attested copies) and the appropriate exemption fee. The 2007 fees are £250.

KEY POINTS

- The Part 1 MRCOG examination is held twice every year (March and September) at different centres in the UK and overseas.

- The closing dates for receiving the application forms are 1st December for the March examination and 1st June for the September examination.

- Holding a medical qualification is the only eligibility requirement for the Part 1 examination. Registration as a medical practitioner is no longer required.

- There is no limit to the number of attempts allowed at the Part 1.

- Exemption from the Part 1 may be granted to doctors who have passed certain overseas examinations before 1st January 2007.

- Overseas candidates are advised to pass the Part 1 examination before they come to the UK for training.

- The average pass rate in the Part 1 examination is around 35%, which remains fairly constant for all attempts.

- Statistically speaking, your chances of passing the Part 1 examination are much higher if you take it sooner, rather than later, after graduation.

- The regulations are subject to regular review. Application forms and further information on the latest examination regulations, fees and venues can be obtained from the College website at *http://www.rcog.org.uk*. Another useful source of information is the MRCOG Blog (*http://web.mac.com/k.sharif*).

2

Syllabus and Preparation

Introduction

The regulations for the Part 1 examination state '…the examination embraces those subjects which form part of the general education of any specialist and particularly those aspects which are applicable to obstetrics and gynaecology'. The Examination Committee of the RCOG has published a syllabus that defines the subjects included in the examination. The phrase 'comprehensive knowledge' is liberally used in the syllabus to describe the depth of knowledge required. The fact that almost 70% of candidates fail the Part 1 examination indicates that the majority either do not understand the scope of the examination or find difficulties in reaching the required standards. In this chapter we will first present the syllabus for the Part 1, then discuss how to achieve the required standards.

Syllabus for the Part 1 Examination

Anatomy

Comprehensive knowledge of the regional anatomy of the pelvis, abdomen, thorax, breast, endocrine glands, hypothalamus, spinothalamic tracts and meninges. Detailed knowledge of relevant bones, joints, muscles, blood vessels, lymphatics, nerve supply and histology. Basic understanding of cell structure.

Embryology

Comprehensive knowledge of gametogenesis and fertilization, of organogenesis and the development of the embryo in all body systems, of the development of placenta, membranes and amniotic fluid and of structural changes in the newborn.

Statistics and Epidemiology

Understanding of commonly used terms and techniques. Interpretation of results of research investigations.

Endocrinology

Comprehensive knowledge of all hormones and humoral agents (both sexes) including their formation from precursors, storage, release, transport, mode and site of action, regulation and distribution in all body compartments as well as their physiological and pathological activities.

Microbiology

Comprehensive knowledge of the characteristics, recognition, prevention, eradication and pathological effects of all commonly encountered bacteria, viruses, Rickettsia, fungi, protozoa, parasites and toxins, including an understanding of the principles of infection control.

Immunology

Comprehensive knowledge of the immune mechanism, both cell-mediated and humorally mediated, and of the principles of reproductive immunology, graft-host interaction, immunization, immunosuppression, allergies and anaphylactic reactions.

Pharmacology

Comprehensive knowledge of properties, pharmacodynamics, actions, interactions and hazards of drugs and anaesthetics agents commonly used in the mother, fetus and neonate. Detailed knowledge of the principles of teratogenicity and of prescribing during pregnancy and lactation.

Physiology

Comprehensive knowledge of human physiology with particular reference to the male and female reproductive systems, pregnancy, the fetus and the neonate. Quantitative information about common physiological activities. Understanding of the principles of nutrition, water, electrolyte and acid-base balance and cell biology.

Pathology

Comprehensive knowledge of general pathological principles including general, tissue and cellular responses to trauma, infection, inflammation, therapeutic intervention (especially by the use of irradiation, cytotoxic drugs and hormones), disturbances in blood flow, loss of body fluids and neoplasia. Detailed knowledge of common pathological conditions.

Genetics

Understanding of the structure and function of chromosomes and genes. Knowledge of the principles of inheritance of chromosomal and genetic disorders. Detailed knowledge of common inherited disorders and of common fetal malformations.

Biochemistry

Comprehensive knowledge of the metabolism of carbohydrates, lipids, proteins and nucleic acids, of the roles of vitamins, minerals and enzymes and of the composition and regulation of intracellular and extracellular fluids. Detailed knowledge of the processes involved in steroidogenesis, placental function and materno-fetal interactions.

Biophysics

Knowledge of the physical principles and biological effects of heat, sound and electromagnetic radiation. Understanding of the principles of laser, electrocardiography, isotopes, X-rays, ultrasound and magnetic resonance imaging.

▌ Preparation

Reading

The first problem facing prospective Part 1 candidates is deciding on a realistic and suitable reading list. The difficulty is in choosing between relatively small books (with the concern that they may not be adequate for the examination) and large volumes that are difficult to master and know well. Most candidates will be preparing for the examination during busy junior hospital posts that do not lend themselves adequately to memorizing very large volumes of basic science textbooks.

Unfortunately, the luxury of whole weeks and months dedicated solely to studying does not exist after leaving medical school.

Candidates are further confused when some suggested reading lists, which include *Gray's Anatomy*, *Walter and Israel's Pathology* and Topley and Wilson's *Microbiology*, go on to say that these books may not be enough for the Part 1 examination! This cautious attitude, however understandable, is not much help to candidates. A more realistic approach is to read well one of the smaller books written specifically for the Part 1 MRCOG. Then if there is anything that you do not understand well or that you have found from MCQ books to be a common question in Part 1, you could look it up in a larger textbook.

A good tip is to start preparing for the Part 1 as soon as possible after graduation. This will ensure that the basic sciences you have studied as an undergraduate are still up-to-date and fresh in your mind (or at least fresher than they will be a few years later). We suggest a minimum of 6–9 months for preparation.

Obstetrics and Gynaecology Basic Science Textbooks

Read one of the general basic science textbooks that are specific for obstetrics and gynaecology. These have been written with the Part 1 MRCOG in mind and contain knowledge pertinent to both the content and the format of the examination. They also come in small readable sizes.

An important point to note is that these books are *very* condensed. All the knowledge in them (including tables and diagrams) is essential to remember. It is far better to study a small book well rather than a large book badly.

Two basic science textbooks which are particularly popular among the Part 1 candidates are:

- de Swiet M, Chamberlain GVP and Bennett P (2001) *Basic Science in Obstetrics and Gynaecology – A Textbook for MRCOG Part 1*, 3rd edition, Edinburgh: Churchill Livingstone.
- Chard T and Lilford R (1997) *Basic Sciences for Obstetrics and Gynaecology*, 5th edition, London: Springer-Verlag.

These are only two examples and many other books, not mentioned here, are also suitable for studying for the Part 1 examination. You should always use the latest edition of any book.

General Basic Science Textbooks

Having read your obstetrics and gynaecology basic science textbook *well*, you should use the remainder of your preparation time to read general basic science textbooks. Which books to read is generally a matter of personal choice. We recommend the books you have read as an undergraduate (their latest editions) as you will be more familiar with their styles. With regard to what to read in these books, this will depend mainly on two factors. First, you should read about what you have not clearly understood from your main book. Second, you should read further about the topics of the syllabus not covered well in your main book. In our experience, anatomy and pathology are two subjects that usually require further reading.

The RCOG bookshop (*http://www.rcog.org.uk/index.asp?PageID=73*) has a regularly updated list of textbooks suitable for the Part 1 preparation. You are well advised to look through the bookshop's web page when you start preparing.

Multiple-Choice Question Books

Practising **multiple-choice questions** (MCQ) should form a major part of your preparation. This is as important as reading textbooks, and will be discussed further in Chapter 4. Many MCQ books have been written specifically for the Part 1 examination and contain not only exam-like questions but also explanatory answers. These books are very good for both self-assessment and revision. These can also be found on the RCOG bookshop web page.

MRCOG Courses

A common question asked by many Part 1 candidates is: do I need to attend a course before taking the Part 1? The answer is a qualified 'yes'. This means that if you are able to attend a course, then you should. Courses provide many benefits. They focus your mind on the task of passing the exam; draw your attention to certain important points in the syllabus that might otherwise have escaped you; allow you to practise in a supervised environment where immediate feedback enhances learning and the retention of facts; put you together with other doctors who have similar aims (a common-predicament support group); and give you the opportunity to draw on the experience of the course tutors, who are usually experienced consultants and trainers.

Having said that, it is important to choose your course wisely, just as you choose your books wisely. The best indicator of course quality is how long it has been running for, the seniority and experience of the tutors (these tend to go hand in hand), and most importantly the comments of other candidates who have attended the course previously. Another consideration, particularly for overseas candidates, is geographical location. It is very expensive to come to the UK just to attend a Part 1 course. The RCOG publishes on its website dates and locations of MRCOG courses (*http://www.rcog.org.uk/index.asp?PageID=104*). Also the *MRCOG Survival Courses* (*http://www.mrcogcourses.co.uk*) have been organizing courses for over 10 years and run very popular MRCOG Part 1 intensive courses in London, Birmingham, Dubai and India on a regular basis.

Web Resources

Not infrequently during your Part 1 preparation you may run into a difficult question to which you cannot find the answer or you may have a query about the exam system or regulations. With the availability of the internet and e-mails, the answers should be easily available if you know where to look and whom to ask.

With regard to questions and basic science facts, your first port of call (after your textbooks) should be Google (*http://www.google.com*). This popular general search engine is a very good source of medical resources. If you still do not find your answer, try the MRCOG Blog (*http://web.mac.com/k.sharif/iWeb*), which is a blogging site for MRCOG facts, questions, regulations etc.

With regard to exam system and regulations queries, you should first try the RCOG (*http://www.rcog.org.uk*), and if you still require further help, try the MRCOG Blog (*http://web.mac.com/k.sharif/iWeb*).

KEY POINTS

- The topics covered in the Part 1 MRCOG examination are basic sciences as applied to obstetrics and gynaecology. These include anatomy, physiology, biochemistry, endocrinology, genetics, pathology, microbiology, immunology, pharmacology and statistics.

- Start preparing for the Part 1 examination as soon as possible after graduation.

- First read a basic science textbook specifically written for obstetrics and gynaecology.

- You should also supplement your knowledge by reading general basic science textbooks. Your undergraduate books are generally recommended.

- Practising MCQ is as important as reading textbooks.

- A suggested reading list is provided at the RCOG website (*http://www. rcog.org.uk*).

- Useful internet resources can be found at:

  - *http://www.rcog.org.uk*
  - *http://www.mrcogcourses.co.uk*
  - *http://web.mac.com/k.sharif/iWeb*
  - *http://www.google.com*

3

The Examination System

Introduction

The format of the Part 1 examination has undergone many changes since it was first introduced in 1970. Initially, the examination consisted of an essay paper and a multiple-choice question (MCQ) paper. In 1978 the essay paper was abolished and in 1982 another MCQ paper was added. At different stages there were suggestions of adding an oral component, similar to the Primary Examination of the Fellowship of the Royal College of Surgeons (FRCS). For practical reasons, these suggestions were not adopted and are unlikely to be adopted in the foreseeable future. Despite numerous recent changes in the Part 2 examination format, the current Part 1 format has not changed and is set to stay for many years to come. Understanding the examination system will aid intelligent preparation and maximize the chances of success.

The MCQ Papers

The examination consists of two MCQ papers, each containing 60 questions (every MCQ has one opening statement followed by five responses – see below). One paper is taken during the morning and the other during the afternoon of the same day. Two hours are allowed for each paper.

The questions in the two papers are divided into sections, each addressing a different topic of the syllabus. The exact arrangement may vary between different examinations, but the following is common:

Paper 1

- 20 MCQ on anatomy and embryology (18 and 2 respectively)

- 20 MCQ on endocrinology and statistics/epidemiology (18 and 2 respectively)
- 20 MCQ on microbiology and pharmacology

Paper 2

- 20 MCQ on physiology
- 20 MCQ on pathology, genetics and immunology
- 20 MCQ on biochemistry and biophysics

It is important to know this information when planning your final revision. As you will see later in this chapter, you do not need to pass in every section in the examination. Provided that your total mark is equal to or above the pass mark, you will pass. A useful tip, if you have limited time for revision before the examination, is to spend more time revising subjects with more questions rather than those with fewer questions.

▌ The MCQ Format

Each MCQ in the Part 1 examination consists of an opening statement (stem) followed by five items (branches) identified by the letters A to E. The stem is usually a brief, clear and unambiguous statement addressing an important topic. Each of the items could be either true or false. The questions look like the following example:

1. Adrenaline:
   A. is a vasoconstrictor.
   B. is lipolytic.
   C. increases glucose output from the liver.
   D. is synthesized from noradrenaline.
   E. is excreted as glucoronide conjugate.

In the actual examination you will be provided with a computer answer sheet, a special grade HB pencil and a rubber. The answer sheet contains a row of five boxes for each question and is numbered accordingly. Each box refers to a single item. In each box there are two lozenges labelled **T** (true) and **F** (false). You will be required to indicate whether you knew a particular item to be true or false by blacking out in **bold** either the 'true' or 'false' lozenge. The whole lozenge should be blacked out. Other marks such as ✗ or ✓ are not recognized by the computer.

You must use only the grade HB pencil provided for completing all parts of the answer sheets. This is essential as the answer sheets are marked by a computer which is programmed to recognize the shade of this pencil mark.

It is important to mark an answer for each branch (by blacking out one lozenge). If you make a mistake and want to change an answer, you should use the provided rubber to erase it. Erasures should be left clean, with no smudges.

A few weeks before the examination date you will receive detailed instructions from the RCOG on how to complete the answer sheet. You are strongly advised to read these instructions thoroughly and acquaint yourself with their details. The examination hall is not the ideal place to be reading answering instructions for the first time. Detailed instructions and sample answer sheet for the MCQ papers in the Part 1 examination are provided in Appendix 3.

The Marking System

The answer sheets are marked by computer. Each item correctly answered (whether it is 'true' or 'false') is awarded one mark (+1). For each incorrect answer no marks are awarded or deducted (0).

The marks of the 600 items (2 papers × 60 MCQ × 5 items) are added up by the computer and the total mark is expressed as a percentage.

The next step in the marking system is a computer-based detailed analysis of the results to decide the pass mark. This analysis takes into account the general performance of the candidates as well as their performance in specific *marker* questions. These are questions that have been well tried in previous examinations and can discriminate between the weaker and the stronger candidates. Based on this analysis, the Examination Committee then decides on the pass mark. Candidates whose total mark reaches or exceeds this mark will pass, regardless of their performance in individual sections of the papers.

The Pass Mark and Pass Rate

The pass mark is usually around 80%. On average, one out of three candidates will pass (average 35%–37%).

▌ The Results

Approximately 6 weeks after the examination the results are announced. Your result will be sent to you by first class mail (air mail if your correspondence address is abroad). The list of the successful candidates is available on the College website (from about 18:00 h on the day of the results) as well as being displayed on the notice board in the College front hall (from 12:00 h).

Congratulations are due to successful candidates. Their next step is the Part 2 examination and Chapter 15 in this book will guide them.

Unsuccessful candidates will undoubtedly be very disappointed. They are to be reminded that many Members of the RCOG have not passed on the first attempt. The Examination Department of the RCOG considers it essential to inform unsuccessful candidates in which topics they have failed. In fact, this was the original reason behind dividing the examination in 1982 into two papers, each containing different sections addressing specific topics. Unsuccessful candidates are currently informed of the grade (borderline or fail) obtained in the sections they have failed. This valuable information should help guide their future preparation.

KEY POINTS

- The Part 1 MRCOG examination consists of two MCQ papers, each containing 60 questions. Two hours are allowed for each paper. The questions are divided into different sections, each addressing a particular topic of the syllabus.

- Each MCQ consists of a stem and five branches. Your answer to each branch is either true 'T' or false 'F'.

- Each item correctly answered (whether it is 'true' or 'false') is awarded one mark (+1). For each incorrect answer, no marks are awarded or deducted (0).

- After detailed analysis of the general performance in the examination as well as the performance in special marker questions the pass mark is decided.

- The pass mark is usually 80% and the pass rate about 35%.

- Candidates whose total mark is equal to or above the pass mark will pass, regardless of their performance in individual sections of the papers.

- The results will be announced six weeks after the examination.

- Unsuccessful candidates will be informed in which topics of the syllabus they have failed. This information should help them in future preparation.

4

Multiple-Choice Question Techniques

Introduction

Multiple-choice questions (MCQ) are widely used in both under-graduate and postgraduate medical examinations. They provide a reliable and valid method of testing factual information as well as covering a wide range of topics. Furthermore, their computer-marking is totally objective and eliminates any element of examiners' bias. In addition to factual knowledge (which is essential for all examinations), there are certain tips that can improve your performance in MCQ. In the current jargon, these tips are called 'MCQ techniques'. In this chapter we will first describe briefly how MCQ are set and then discuss these 'techniques' in detail.

Setting MCQ

Contrary to the popular belief among candidates, setting MCQ is as difficult as answering them. Some examiners will go even further and claim it is more difficult! The questions are set by a panel of experienced examiners, and are thoroughly scrutinized and re-scrutinized before being included in the examination. Every question should be as clear and brief as possible. It should address an important and common subject relevant to the syllabus. The answer should be factual information that lends itself to the 'true/false' format and could be found in standard textbooks. Debatable issues and mutually exclusive options are avoided. The difficulty in setting MCQ is finding statements that appear plausible but are false. All textbooks mention the true answers and it is far more difficult for examiners to find false statements that do not appear obvious. As setting new MCQ is such a difficult and time-consuming task, the RCOG does not publish all previous examination questions and candidates are not allowed to take the examination papers outside the examination hall.

How to Deal with MCQ

Read Carefully and Understand Clearly

Read the question carefully and make sure you understand it. Do not simply *think* you understand it. When you have to go through 300 items in 2 hours it is not uncommon to rush in and misread the questions. 'Adrenaline' could be easily misread as 'noradrenaline', 'oxy-haemoglobin' as 'carboxy-haemoglobin' and 'fetal haemoglobin' as 'fetal blood'. In every question, the opening stem should be read together with each of the options (A–E) and taken as a single item. Each item should be considered independently of the other statements.

Do not Read between the Lines

Accept the question at face value and do not look for catches or hidden meanings. Trust that the examiners are trying to test your factual knowledge, not to trick you into making mistakes. What you clearly understand from the question is what is meant by it.

To Guess or not to Guess

After reading (and understanding) each item, your initial response will fall into one of three categories.

First, you may be sure of the answer and have no doubt about the correct response (whether true or false) – go ahead and without hesitation answer the question.

Second, there are those items about which you are not quite certain and yet they 'ring a bell'. You may not immediately know the answer, but from your basic knowledge you could reason it out from first principles – go for it and play your hunches. Such educated hunches that are based on sound judgement and reasoning are more often right than wrong, and you are advised to be bold and answer these items accordingly.

Third, you may be totally ignorant of the answer. The usual advice in such situations, with the *negative* marking system used in many MCQ examinations, is not to guess. However, in the Part 1 MRCOG examination this system has not been used since 1994. There is nothing to be lost by blindly guessing the answers to such items. If you are incorrect you will not lose any marks and if you are correct (50% probability) you will gain. Readers who are preparing for other examinations that still use the negative marking system should not guess blindly.

What is the Pass Mark?

At the time of your examination nobody knows the answer to this question, not even the examiners. As we have seen in the previous chapter, the Part 1 is a norm-referenced examination where the performance of all the candidates has to be analysed before the pass mark is decided. It is, therefore, wrong to assume that there is a 'safe' score, count your responses until you reach it and then stop. You should aim to score as high as possible.

Organize your Time

In the Part 1 MRCOG examination you are allowed 2 hours for every paper (60 questions), which translates into 2 minutes per question (5 items) or 24 seconds per item. This might appear too little, but it is not. The items you are sure of will take only a few seconds. The same applies to those items about which you are totally ignorant. We suggest you go through the whole paper first, answering those questions to which you are sure you know the answers. As you are unlikely to change these answers, you are advised to record them on the answer sheet from the outset. The remaining time should be directed to the unanswered, more time-consuming items about which you are uncertain but have enough basic knowledge to make reasoned hunches. You should have marked these items on the question paper during your first reading to facilitate coming back to them. Any remaining time should be spent on revising the answers, but remember that your first thought is likely to be the correct answer.

Fill-in the Answer Sheet Correctly

A sure recipe for disaster in MCQ examinations is to make a systematic error in recording the answers. If you answer question 1 in place of question 2, all the following answers will also be recorded wrongly. Such mistakes are quite easily done under the stress of the examination. Make sure when you fill-in every answer that it is in the right place.

MCQ Terminology

Candidates may find difficulty in understanding some words commonly used in MCQ. The following is a guide to the accepted meanings of some of these troublesome words:

- Common/characteristic/usual/typical: what is expected to be found in the average, textbook description.
- Recognized/may occur/can occur: has been described, even if rarely.
- Essential feature: must occur to make a diagnosis.
- Frequently/often: imply a rate of occurrence greater than 50%.
- Never: 0%.
- Always: 100%.
- Rare: < 5%.

Beware that absolutes are very rare in medicine. Items that contain always or never are often false.

Practising MCQ

This is as important as reading textbooks and should form 50% of your preparation. Practising MCQ will familiarize you with the examination system and help identify areas of weakness in your knowledge. Some MCQ books (written specifically for the Part 1 candidates) are listed in Chapter 2. Other basic science MCQ books will also be useful. You should use these for self-assessment (i.e. attempt to answer the questions before looking at the provided answers). The practice and experience you will gain in reasoning and educated hunches will go a long way to maximize your score in the actual examination.

KEY POINTS

- The Part 1 examination questions are clear and brief, address important and common subjects and test factual non-controversial knowledge.

- When answering MCQ, read the stem and each option carefully, understand them clearly and consider them independently of other options.

- Take each question at its face value.

- Work out the answers by educated reasoning from basic principles.

- If you do not know the answer, guess. There is no negative marking system in the Part 1 examination. If you guess an answer there is (at least theoretically) a 50% chance of getting it right, and nothing to lose.

- Aim to score as high as possible and do not assume that there is a safe score above which you do not need to attempt any more questions.

- Mark your answers clearly and accurately and keep an eye on the time.

Anatomy

5

ANATOMY: QUESTIONS

1. Contents of the rectus sheath include:

    A. the external oblique muscle.

    B. the inferior epigastric artery.

    C. the subcostal nerve.

    D. the pyramidalis muscle.

    E. the musculophrenic artery.

2. The inferior vena cava:

    A. is joined by the left ovarian vein.

    B. is retroperitoneal.

    C. lies behind the third part of the duodenum.

    D. pierces the diaphragm through the same opening as the azygos vein.

    E. lies in front of the medial border of the right psoas major muscle.

3. The inferior epigastric artery:

    A. lies lateral to the deep inguinal ring.

    B. originates from the internal iliac artery.

    C. anastomoses with a branch of the internal thoracic artery.

    D. pierces the fascia transversalis.

    E. passes in front of the arcuate line.

4. Boundaries of the femoral ring include:

    A. the femoral vein.

    B. the femoral artery.

C. the lacunar ligament.

D. the inguinal ligament.

E. the pectineal ligament.

5. **Muscles attached to the perineal body include:**

A. bulbo-spongiosus muscle.

B. ischio-cavernosus muscle.

C. external anal sphincter.

D. deep transverse perineal muscle.

E. pubo-coccygeus part of the levator ani muscle.

6. **Following ligation of the internal iliac artery, collateral circulation is established through anastomosis between:**

A. inferior vesical and superior vesical arteries.

B. superior gluteal and inferior gluteal arteries.

C. uterine and ovarian arteries.

D. middle haemorrhoidal and superior haemorrhoidal arteries.

E. ilio-lumbar and lumbar arteries.

7. **In the female breast:**

A. the areola and nipple overlie a pad of fat.

B. each lactiferous duct drains a group of lobes.

C. the alveoli have a rich nerve supply.

D. malignancy spreads to the vertebrae through lymphatic channels.

E. the lymph capillaries anastomose with those of the anterior abdominal wall.

8. **The female breast:**

A. is mesodermal in origin.

B. overlies the serratus anterior muscle.

C. consists of 15–25 lobes.

D. extends from the 2nd to the 6th rib in the midclavicular line.

E. has lymphatic connection between both sides.

9. The spinal subarachnoid space:

    A. contains cerebro-spinal fluid.

    B. is traversed by the ligamentum denticulatum.

    C. terminates at the level of the fifth lumbar vertebra.

    D. is crossed by fibrous processes connecting the pia mater to the arachnoid mater.

    E. communicates with the subarachnoid space of the posterior cranial fossa.

10. The right uterine artery:

    A. is a branch of the internal iliac artery.

    B. crosses under the ureter.

    C. anastomoses with the ovarian artery in the broad ligament.

    D. runs along the anterior surface of the body of the uterus.

    E. passes through the deep inguinal ring.

11. The lumbar vertebra has:

    A. the foramen transversarium in the transverse process.

    B. an articular facet at the tip of the transverse process.

    C. three primary centres of ossification.

    D. medial and lateral rotatory movement.

    E. the multifidus muscle attached to the mamillary process.

12. After birth:

    A. the intra-abdominal part of the left umbilical vein becomes the ligamentum teres of the liver.

    B. the ductus arteriosus becomes the ligamentum arteriosum.

    C. the urachus becomes the median umbilical ligament.

    D. the distal part of the umbilical artery becomes the medial umbilical ligament.

    E. the proximal part of the umbilical artery becomes the superior vesical artery.

13. The Bartholin's gland:

    A. is the homologue of the prostate in the male.

    B. lies superficial to the perineal membrane.

    C. has a duct which is lined with transitional epithelium.

    D. lies deep to the bulbo-spongiosus muscle.

    E. is normally palpable.

14. The pituitary gland:

    A. is extra-dural.

    B. when enlarged can cause binasal hemianopia.

    C. is ectodermal in origin.

    D. lies above the diaphragma sellae.

    E. lies medial to the cavernous sinuses.

15. The vagina:

    A. is lined with non-keratinized stratified squamous epithelium.

    B. is directed upwards and backwards.

    C. normally has a pH of 4–5 during child-bearing years.

    D. has abundant mucous-secreting cells.

    E. has a posterior wall longer than its anterior wall.

16. Connections between the portal and the systemic venous circulations include anastomosis between:

    A. the oesophageal branches of the left gastric vein and the oesophageal branches of the azygos vein.

    B. the superior rectal vein and the middle and inferior rectal veins.

    C. the right colic vein and the right renal vein.

    D. the left renal vein and the left suprarenal vein.

    E. the superior mesenteric vein and the inferior vena cava.

17. The transpyloric plane passes at the level:

    A. of the second lumbar vertebra.

    B. of the fundus of the gall bladder.

    C. at which the superior mesenteric artery comes off the aorta.

    D. of the tip of the tenth costal cartilage.

    E. just above the hilum of the right kidney.

18. Lymph nodes draining the abdominal wall include:

    A. intercostal nodes.

    B. superficial inguinal nodes.

    C. para-aortic nodes.

    D. mediastinal nodes.

    E. axillary nodes.

19. Retroperitoneal structures include the:

    A. spleen.

    B. pancreas.

    C. uterus.

    D. aorta.

    E. ureter.

20. In the newborn baby the:

    A. mandible is in two halves.

    B. anterior fontanelle lies between two frontal and two parietal bones.

    C. spinal cord extends to the level of the fifth lumbar vertebra.

    D. urinary bladder lies in the abdomen.

    E. mastoid process is well developed.

21. The anterior wall of the rectus sheath:

    A. is adherent to the rectus abdominis muscle at the tendinous intersections.

    B. ends inferiorly at the arcuate line.

    C. above the costal margin is formed of the aponeuroses of the external and internal oblique muscles.

    D. overlies the pyramidalis muscle.

    E. is pierced by the superior epigastric artery.

22. The anterior spinal artery:

    A. is a branch of the internal carotid artery.

    B. anastomoses with the posterior spinal arteries at the conus medullaris.

C. anastomoses with the spinal branch of the eleventh intercostal artery.

D. is smaller than the posterior spinal artery.

E. is the only vessel supplying the anterior part of the cervical spinal cord.

23. **The pleura:**

A. extends into the interlobar clefts of the lungs.

B. extends above the clavicle.

C. is continuous throughout its parietal and visceral layers.

D. over the domes of the diaphragm is supplied by the phrenic nerve.

E. lies behind the upper pole of the kidney.

24. **The pudendal nerve:**

A. is derived from the ventral rami of the 2nd, 3rd and 4th sacral nerves.

B. passes between the piriformis and the coccygeus muscles.

C. passes through the lesser sciatic foramen.

D. passes through the greater sciatic foramen.

E. lies on the medial wall of the ischio-rectal fossa.

25. **The inguinal ligament is situated in front of:**

A. the external iliac artery.

B. the iliacus muscle.

C. the ilio-inguinal nerve.

D. the femoral nerve.

E. the internal oblique muscle.

26. **The superficial inguinal ring:**

A. is triangular in shape.

B. is situated below the pubic tubercle.

C. contains the round ligament of the uterus in the female.

D. contains the external spermatic fascia in the male.

E. lies opposite the deep inguinal ring.

27. The conjoint tendon:

    A. lies in front of the lacunar ligament.

    B. is attached to the pectineal line behind the attachment of the inguinal ligament.

    C. forms part of the posterior wall of the inguinal canal.

    D. is attached to the pubic crest.

    E. lies in front of the spermatic cord.

28. The cremaster muscle:

    A. surrounds the round ligament of the uterus in the female.

    B. is supplied by a branch of the inferior epigastric artery.

    C. is formed of fibres from the external oblique muscle.

    D. is attached to the pubic tubercle.

    E. is supplied by the genital branch of the genito-femoral nerve.

29. The left adrenal gland:

    A. at birth is nearly as large as the kidney.

    B. lies on the left crus of the diaphragm.

    C. lies behind the tail of the pancreas.

    D. is partially covered with the spleen.

    E. forms part of the stomach bed.

30. Branches of the inferior mesenteric artery include:

    A. the superior gluteal artery.

    B. the sigmoid artery.

    C. the upper left colic artery.

    D. the superior rectal artery.

    E. the inferior gluteal artery.

31. The fascia transversalis:

    A. is pierced by the inferior epigastric artery.

    B. is continuous with the fascia iliaca.

    C. is continuous with Colles' fascia.

    D. is continuous with the diaphragmatic fascia.

    E. forms the posterior wall of the femoral sheath.

32. The ilio-inguinal nerve:
    A. passes behind the kidney.
    B. arises from the posterior ramus of the first lumbar nerve.
    C. supplies the skin over the mons pubis in the female.
    D. supplies the skin of the anterior third of the scrotum in the male.
    E. emerges from the superficial inguinal ring.

33. The major supports of the uterus include:
    A. the levator ani muscle.
    B. the utero-sacral ligament.
    C. the round ligament.
    D. the pubo-cervical ligament.
    E. the infundibulo-pelvic ligament.

34. The quadratus lumborum muscle:
    A. lies behind the lateral arcuate ligament.
    B. is inserted in the lateral half of the lower border of the twelfth rib.
    C. acts to cause lateral rotation of the lumbar vertebrae.
    D. is supplied by the twelfth thoracic nerve.
    E. originates from the ilio-lumbar ligament.

35. The dartos muscle:
    A. acts to elevate the testis.
    B. lies superficial to Colles' fascia.
    C. is supplied by sympathetic fibres.
    D. is attached to the skin.
    E. is a striated muscle.

36. The gubernaculum:
    A. is endodermal in origin.
    B. passes through the inguinal canal.
    C. forms the ovarian ligament.
    D. has a retroperitoneal course.
    E. is attached to the labium minus.

37. The inguinal canal:

    A. lies above the lateral half of the inguinal ligament.

    B. has an internal opening which is medial to the inferior epigastric artery.

    C. transmits the round ligament of the uterus in the female.

    D. has a posterior wall which is formed exclusively by the fascia transversalis.

    E. transmits the abnormal obturator artery.

38. A direct inguinal hernia:

    A. passes through the deep inguinal ring.

    B. may descend into the scrotum.

    C. has a neck which lies medial to the inferior epigastric artery.

    D. may pass through the superficial inguinal ring.

    E. is always acquired.

39. The femoral sheath:

    A. contains the femoral nerve.

    B. has an anterior wall which is an extension of the external oblique aponeurosis.

    C. has its anterior wall pierced by the femoral branch of the genito-femoral nerve.

    D. has a posterior wall which is an extension of the fascia iliaca.

    E. contains the femoral artery.

40. The coverings of the spermatic cord:

    A. extend down to cover the testis.

    B. are supplied by the first and second sacral nerves.

    C. have lymphatic drainage to the external iliac lymph nodes.

    D. are in three layers below the superficial inguinal ring.

    E. have the same arterial supply as the vas deferens.

41. The vas deferens:

    A. lies medial to the epididymis.

    B. lies lateral to the seminal vesicle.

    C. has a retroperitoneal course.

    D. is about 45 cm long.

    E. crosses over the external iliac vessels.

42. The lymphatic drainage of:

    A. the epididymis is to para-aortic lymph nodes.

    B. the testis is to the inguinal lymph nodes.

    C. the cervix is to the internal iliac lymph nodes.

    D. the kidney is to the external iliac lymph nodes.

    E. the vulva is to the deep femoral lymph node of Cloquet.

43. Embryological remnants of the mesonephric tubules in the male include:

    A. the appendix testis.

    B. the appendix of epididymis.

    C. the paradidymis.

    D. the utriculus masculinus.

    E. the ductulus aberrans superior.

44. The falciform ligament:

    A. contains the ligamentum teres of the liver in its lower border.

    B. is attached to the upper surface of the liver in the midline.

    C. is attached to the central tendon of the diaphragm.

    D. connects the spleen to the liver.

    E. is attached to the linea alba.

45. The epiploic foramen:

    A. connects the lesser sac to the greater sac of the peritoneum.

    B. lies above the second part of the duodenum.

    C. lies in front of the inferior vena cava.

    D. lies behind the hepatic vein.

    E. lies below the caudate process of the liver.

46. The bare area of the liver is:

    A. in contact with the right adrenal gland.

    B. bound by the coronary ligament.

C. bound by the porta hepatis.

D. in contact with the portal vein.

E. in contact with the diaphragm.

47. **Structures related to the posterior surface of the stomach include:**

A. the head of the pancreas.

B. the left adrenal gland.

C. the splenic artery.

D. the jejunum.

E. the transverse colon.

48. **The thyroid gland:**

A. is fixed to the 2nd, 3rd and 4th rings of the trachea.

B. develops from the cranial end of the thyro-glossal duct.

C. is supplied by sympathetic vasoconstrictor fibres.

D. extends along the side of the trachea as low as the sixth tracheal ring.

E. is completely adherent to the pretracheal fascia.

49. **Structures enclosed within the pretracheal fascia include:**

A. the recurrent laryngeal nerve.

B. the thyroid gland.

C. the parathyroid gland.

D. the omo-hyoid muscle.

E. the main trunk of the inferior thyroid artery.

50. **The internal anal sphincter:**

A. is under voluntary control.

B. extends down to Hilton's white line.

C. is innervated from the inferior hypogastric plexus.

D. is capable of maintaining continence of flatus and faeces on its own.

E. contracts in response to sympathetic stimulation.

51. The part of the anal canal below Hilton's white line:

    A. is ectodermal in origin.

    B. has arterial supply which anastomoses with the arteries of the anal canal above Hilton's line.

    C. has venous drainage to the portal venous system.

    D. drains to the superficial inguinal lymph nodes.

    E. has somatic supply from the inferior rectal nerve.

52. The superior rectal artery:

    A. crosses the left ureter.

    B. has rich anastomosis with the inferior rectal artery.

    C. is the direct continuation of the inferior mesenteric artery.

    D. supplies the mucous membrane of the rectum and anal canal above Hilton's line.

    E. runs along the root of the pelvic mesocolon.

53. Structures situated posterior to the superior mesenteric artery include:

    A. the neck of the pancreas.

    B. the right ureter.

    C. the left renal vein.

    D. the second part of duodenum.

    E. the right ovarian artery.

54. The femoral triangle:

    A. is bound by the medial border of the sartorius muscle.

    B. is bound by the medial border of the adductor longus muscle.

    C. is bound by the inguinal ligament.

    D. has the adductor longus muscle in its floor.

    E. has the rectus femoris muscle in its floor.

55. In the human kidney:

    A. the distal convoluted tubules lie in the medulla.

    B. the renal vein lies in front of the renal artery in the hilum.

    C. the renal pelvis is lined with transitional epithelium.

    D. the anterior surface is completely covered by peritoneum.

    E. abnormal renal arteries may be associated with hydronephrosis.

56. Structures passing through the lesser sciatic foramen include:

    A. the pudendal nerve.

    B. the sciatic nerve.

    C. the tendon of the obturator internus muscle.

    D. the inferior gluteal nerve.

    E. the posterior cutaneous nerve of the thigh.

57. The ureter:

    A. is about 25 cm in length.

    B. lies on the lateral edge of the psoas major muscle.

    C. is endodermal in origin.

    D. lies in front of the renal artery at the hilum of the kidney.

    E. receives some of its blood supply from the ovarian artery.

58. The right ureter lies posterior to:

    A. the ischial spine.

    B. the ovarian artery.

    C. the vas deferens.

    D. the genito-femoral nerve.

    E. the third part of the duodenum.

59. The trigone of the urinary bladder:

    A. is the most distensible part of the bladder.

    B. lies between the internal urethral orifice and the orifices of the ureters.

    C. is covered with transitional epithelium which has abundant glands.

    D. overlies the vagina in the female.

    E. has an internal elevation (the uvula vesicae) which is caused by the underlying median lobe of the prostate in the male.

60. The urinary bladder:

    A. has a vesical venous plexus which communicates with the vaginal venous plexus.

    B. is supplied by branches from the vaginal artery.

    C. is supplied by sympathetic nervous fibres which stimulate contraction of the detrusor muscle.

    D. embryologically is derived from the urogenital sinus.

    E. is connected to the umbilicus via the lateral ligament of the bladder.

61. In the male urethra:

    A. the sphincter urethrae muscle (external sphincter) is capable of maintaining continence of urine in the absence of action from the internal sphincter.

    B. the ducts of the bulbo-urethral glands open into the membranous urethra.

    C. the prostatic ducts open into the prostatic utricle.

    D. the external urethral meatus is the narrowest part.

    E. embryologically has a mixed endodermal and mesodermal origin.

62. In the normal cervix:

    A. the histological internal os lies above the anatomical internal os.

    B. there is an abrupt transition from columnar to squamous epithelium at the squamo-columnar junction.

    C. is predominantly composed of connective tissue.

    D. has sensory supply through the pelvic parasympathetics (S2, 3 and 4).

    E. there are cyclical changes during the menstrual cycle.

63. The uterus:

    A. is completely covered by peritoneum on the posterior surface of its body.

    B. has sensory sympathetic supply through the hypogastric nerves.

    C. may have lymphatic drainage to the superficial inguinal nodes.

   D. in infancy has the cervix larger than the body.
   E. after menopause has the body shrinking to a greater extent
       than the cervix.

64. The adult left ovary:
   A. has veins which drain into the left renal vein.
   B. is covered with peritoneum.
   C. has lymphatic drainage to the internal iliac nodes.
   D. has referred pain along the cutaneous distribution of the
       obturator nerve.
   E. has arterial supply from a branch of the internal iliac
       artery.

65. The ovarian ligament:
   A. is covered by peritoneum.
   B. contains the ovarian vessels.
   C. is attached to the uterus below the attachment of the
       Fallopian tube.
   D. is derived from the gubernaculum.
   E. maintains the ovary in a constant position.

66. The Fallopian tube:
   A. is about 10 cm long.
   B. undergoes atrophic changes after the menopause.
   C. undergoes cyclical changes during the menstrual cycle.
   D. is supplied by a branch of the ovarian artery.
   E. has the same embryological origin as the ovary.

67. The anterior vaginal wall:
   A. is longer than its posterior wall.
   B. is partially covered with peritoneum.
   C. is intimately related to the urethra.
   D. is lined with non-keratinized stratified squamous epithelium
       rich in mucous glands.
   E. normally is in contact with the posterior wall.

68. Contents of the broad ligament include:

A. the Fallopian tube.

B. the paroöphoron.

C. the epoöphoron.

D. the round ligament of the uterus.

E. the ovary.

69. The obturator nerve:

A. arises from the dorsal primary rami of the 2nd, 3rd and 4th lumbar nerves.

B. emerges from the medial side of the psoas major muscle.

C. supplies the obturator internus muscle.

D. passes through the lesser sciatic foramen.

E. is purely motor.

70. Nerves emerging from the lateral border of the psoas major muscle include:

A. the genito-femoral nerve.

B. the ilio-inguinal nerve.

C. the lumbo-sacral trunk.

D. the femoral nerve.

E. the sciatic nerve.

71. In the typical female pelvis:

A. the sacro-iliac joint extends to the lower border of the third piece of the sacrum.

B. the greater sciatic notch is acute.

C. the inferior pubic rami are at a right-angle.

D. in the upright position, the ischial spine and the tip of the coccyx are in the same horizontal plane.

E. the ischial spine lies in the plane of the body of the ischium.

72. In the female pelvis:

A. the symphysis pubis is a primary cartilaginous joint.

B. there are three primary centres of ossification in the innominate bone.

    C. the acetabulum is wholly cartilage at birth.

    D. the posterior cutaneous nerve of the thigh passes through the greater sciatic foramen.

    E. the distance from the pubic tubercle to the acetabular margin is greater than the diameter of the acetabulum.

73. **The levator ani muscle:**

    A. has the origin of its ilio-coccygeus part from the ilium.

    B. acts as a sphincter for the vagina.

    C. forms the medial wall of the ischio-rectal fossa.

    D. takes origin from the posterior surface of the upper border of the body of the pubis.

    E. is innervated by the 2nd, 3rd and 4th sacral nerves.

74. **Branches of the internal iliac artery include:**

    A. the median sacral artery.

    B. the lateral sacral artery.

    C. the superior rectal artery.

    D. the uterine artery.

    E. the superior vesical artery.

75. **The great saphenous vein:**

    A. begins at the medial end of the dorsal venous plexus of the foot.

    B. passes behind the medial malleolus of the tibia.

    C. lies in front of the saphenous nerve.

    D. drains the small saphenous vein.

    E. is joined by the superficial epigastric vein.

76. **The obturator artery:**

    A. is a branch of the internal iliac artery.

    B. passes along the lateral pelvic wall below the obturator nerve.

    C. is replaced by the abnormal obturator artery in less than 3% of people.

    D. gives off a pubic branch which anastomoses with the pubic branch of the superior epigastric artery.

    E. supplies the obturator externus muscle.

77. Contents of the ischio-rectal fossa include the:

    A. perineal branch of the fourth sacral nerve.

    B. pudendal nerve.

    C. inferior rectal artery.

    D. labial nerve.

    E. middle rectal artery.

78. The superficial perineal pouch in the female contains:

    A. the crus of the clitoris.

    B. the Bartholin's gland.

    C. the ischio-cavernosus muscle.

    D. the external urethral sphincter.

    E. the vestibular bulb.

79. Branches of the sacral plexus include:

    A. the femoral nerve.

    B. the lateral cutaneous nerve of the thigh.

    C. the pudendal nerve.

    D. the superior gluteal nerve.

    E. the posterior cutaneous nerve of the thigh.

80. The diaphragm:

    A. is pierced by the greater splanchnic nerve.

    B. has its peritoneal covering supplied exclusively by the phrenic nerve.

    C. is supplied by the phrenic artery which is a branch of the abdominal aorta.

    D. overlies the fundus of the stomach.

    E. actively aids forced expiration.

ANATOMY: ANSWERS

1. BCD

The rectus sheath contains two muscles (rectus abdominis and pyramidalis), four vessels (superior epigastric artery and vein and inferior epigastric artery and vein) and six nerves (lower five intercostal and subcostal nerves).

2. BCE

The inferior vena cava (IVC) is formed by the union of the two common iliac veins behind the right common iliac artery. From there it ascends retroperitoneally in front of the vertebral column to end in the right atrium of the heart. Along its course (from below upwards) it lies behind the root of the mesentery, the third part of the duodenum, the right ovarian (testicular) artery, the head of the pancreas, the first part of the duodenum (from which it is separated by the portal vein and the bile duct), the opening of the lesser sac and the liver. Posteriorly the IVC is related to the right sympathetic trunk and the medial border of the right psoas major muscle. It pierces the right crus of the diaphragm through the same opening as the right phrenic nerve. The azygos vein pierces the diaphragm through the aortic opening. The left ovarian vein drains into the left renal vein.

3. CDE

The inferior epigastric artery is an important anatomical landmark in the anterior abdominal wall and is particularly liable to injury during lateral insertion of the trocar in laparoscopy. It originates from the external iliac artery just above the inguinal ligament. It arises deep to the fascia transversalis, which it pierces as it slants upwards and medially to pass in front of the arcuate line and enter the rectus sheath. At the level of the umbilicus it anastomoses with the superior epigastric artery.

4. ACDE

The femoral ring is the abdominal opening of the femoral canal. Its boundaries are: the pectineal line and pectineal ligament (posteriorly), the femoral vein (laterally), the crescentic edge of the lacunar ligament (medially), and the medial part of the inguinal ligament (anteriorly).

5. ACDE

The perineal body is a fibromuscular mass separating the vulva and the lower vagina from the anal canal. It gives attachment to the following muscles: external anal sphincter bulbo-spongiosus, superficial and deep transverse perineal, and the pubo-coccygeus parts of the levator ani.

6. DE

Ligation of the internal iliac artery is helpful in the management of massive pelvic bleeding as in cases of severe postpartum haemorrhage. For this to be effective, both right and left arteries should be ligated. The long-term blood supply to the pelvic organs is not compromised as adequate collateral circulation is maintained by three anastomoses: between the ilio-lumbar artery (from the posterior division of the internal iliac) and the lumbar artery (from the aorta), between the lateral sacral artery (from the posterior division of the internal iliac) and the median sacral artery (from the aorta), and between the middle haemorrhoidal artery (from the anterior division of the internal iliac) and the superior haemorrhoidal artery (from the inferior mesenteric).

7. E

Please see the explanatory notes in the answer to question 8.

8. BCDE

The breast is ectodermal in origin. It extends from the 2nd to the 6th rib vertically and from the parasternal margin to the midaxillary line horizontally. It is situated in the superficial fascia and overlies the pectoralis major, serratus anterior and external oblique muscles. It consists of 15–25 lobes, each of which drains 20–40 lobules into which 10–100 alveoli drain. Each lobe is drained by a separate lactiferous duct which opens separately into the nipple.

Arterial blood supply is from the internal mammary, lateral thoracic, intercostal and acromio-thoracic arteries. Venous return follows those arteries and is received in the large, mainly valveless veins that also drain the vertebrae; breast malignancy spreads to the bodies of the vertebrae by reflux flow through these veins.

9. ABDE

The spinal cord is surrounded by three meninges: an outer dura, a middle arachnoid and an inner pia. Over the spinal cord the arachnoid is joined to the pia by delicate strands of fibrous tissue that give a cobweb appearance in places, hence the name 'arachnoid'. The pia mater invests the surface of the spinal cord and sends a lateral projection (ligamentum denticulatum) on each side which crosses the subarachnoid space, pierces the arachnoid and is attached to the dura mater. The subarachnoid space extends down to the level of the second sacral vertebra.

10. AC

The uterine artery is a branch of the anterior division of the internal iliac artery. It passes anteriorly and medially on the pelvic floor to reach the lateral aspect of the supravaginal part of the cervix. About 1.5 cm from the cervix it crosses above the ureter (*water under the bridge*) and then turns upwards between the leaves of the broad ligament to run alongside the uterus as far as the entrance of the tube, where it anastomoses with the tubal branch of the ovarian artery.

11. CE

Each vertebra has three primary centres of ossification: the centrum, and the right and left halves of the neural arch. These centres appear by the eighth week of fetal life and are all joined by the third year of life. The most distinctive feature of cervical vertebrae is the presence of foramina transversaria. The thoracic vertebrae have facets at the tip of the transverse processes for articulation with the heads of ribs. The absence of these two features is distinctive of lumbar vertebrae. Movements at the lumbar region include flexion, extension and abduction, but no rotation.

12. ABCDE

Originally there are two umbilical veins in the embryo. As development proceeds, by about day 34 post-fertilization, the right umbilical vein degenerates while the left vein persists.

13. BCD

The Bartholin's (greater vestibular) glands are the homologues of the bulbo-urethral (Cowper's) glands in the male and lie embedded in the posterior parts of the vestibular bulbs just lateral to the vaginal orifice. The gland secretes a mucoid substance during sexual excitement. It is lined with columnar epithelium. Its duct opens lateral to the hymen and demonstrates the common embryological origin of the genital and urinary tracts by being lined with transitional epithelium. The gland is not palpable unless infected.

14. CE

The pituitary gland lies in the pituitary fossa within the sella turcica of the sphenoid bone. The roof of the fossa is made of a fold of dura mater, the diaphragma sellae, which is pierced by the pituitary stalk connecting the gland to the hypothalamus. Superior to the anterior lobe of the pituitary lie the optic chiasma and the optic nerves. A pituitary tumour rising upwards usually passes in front of the chiasma and presses on the medial sides of the optic nerves (fibres from nasal half of the retina) causing bitemporal hemianopia. Anteriorly and posteriorly the gland is related to the intercavernous sinuses; laterally lie the cavernous sinuses with their contents (internal carotid artery and sixth cranial nerve), and inferiorly lie the sphenoidal air sinuses within the body of the sphenoid.

15. ABCE

The vaginal epithelium contains glycogen, which is released when the cells are exfoliated. Döderlein's bacillus, a normal inhabitant, acts upon the glycogen to produce the normal acidity of the vagina. The direction of the vaginal walls is upwards and backwards, a fact that should be remembered when performing digital examination or inserting a speculum. As the cervix enters the vagina through the anterior wall, this is about 2 cm shorter than the posterior wall.

16. ABCE

Other porto-systemic connections include anastomosis between the left colic vein and the left renal vein, the veins of the bare area of the liver and the phrenic veins, as well as the paraumbilical veins connecting the left branch of the portal vein with the superficial veins of the anterior abdominal wall.

17. BCE

The transpyloric plane passes at the level of the first lumbar vertebra, midway between the suprasternal notch and the symphysis pubis. It is important because it defines the position of many viscera. It passes at the level of the pylorus of the stomach and the fundus of the gall bladder, just above the duodeno-jejunal flexure and the hilum of the right kidney, and just below the hilum of the left kidney. It cuts through the costal margin at the tip of the ninth costal cartilage, the upper end of linea semilunaris, the neck of the pancreas and where the spinal cord ends at the conus medullaris.

18. BCDE

The lymphatic drainage of the superficial parts of the abdominal wall above the umbilicus is to the pectoral groups of the axillary nodes and below the umbilicus is to the superficial inguinal nodes. The deeper parts drain into vessels in the transversalis fascia; above the umbilicus these drain into the mediastinal nodes, and below the umbilicus they drain into the external iliac and para-aortic nodes.

19. BDE

Some parts of the alimentary canal lie behind the peritoneum, plastered to the posterior abdominal wall. These include the pancreas, the two ends of the stomach, the duodenum, and the ascending and descending colons. The rectum is also plastered by peritoneum to the hollow of the sacrum. Other retroperitoneal structures include the kidneys, adrenal glands, ureters, aorta, and inferior vena cava.

20. ABD

There are marked differences between the anatomy of the newborn baby and that of the adult. The mandible and the frontal bones are each in two halves. At three months of intrauterine life the spinal cord occupies the whole length of the vertebral column. As development proceeds, the vertebral column grows faster than the spinal cord and at birth the lower end of the cord lies at the level of the third lumbar vertebra. The newborn pelvic cavity is very small and the fundus of the bladder lies in the abdomen. The mastoid process is not well developed and the facial nerve emerges near the lateral surface of the skull and is thus vulnerable to injury at birth.

21. AD

Above the costal margin the anterior wall of the rectus sheath is formed of the aponeurosis of the external oblique only, and there is no true posterior wall. Between the costal margin and midway between the umbilicus and the symphysis pubis the anterior wall is formed of the aponeurosis of the external oblique and the anterior layer of the aponeurosis of the internal oblique, while the posterior wall is formed of the posterior layer of the aponeurosis of the internal oblique and the aponeurosis of the transversus muscle. At that level, the posterior wall ends in the arcuate line, and the aponeuroses of the three muscles (external oblique, internal oblique and transversus) pass in front of the rectus abdominis to form the anterior wall of the sheath.

22. BCE

The anterior spinal artery is formed at the foramen magnum by union of two arteries, one from each vertebral artery. It descends along the anterior median fissure and divides at the conus medullaris into two branches which anastomose with the smaller posterior spinal arteries. The spinal branches of the first and eleventh intercostal arteries (arteries of Adamkiewicz) anastomose with the anterior and posterior spinal arteries and provide an indispensable booster arterial supply. The artery of the eleventh intercostal supplies the spinal cord upwards and downwards. The artery of the first intercostal supplies the cord only downwards from this level. Therefore, the anterior spinal artery provides the only supply for the anterior part of the cervical cord.

23. ABCDE

The pleura is continuous throughout its parietal and visceral layers. The parietal layer lines the thoracic cavity and the upper surface of the diaphragm and the visceral layer invests the surface of the lung, extending into the interlobar clefts. The posterior recess of the pleura extends behind the upper pole of the kidney, an important point to be noted in posterior approaches to the kidney.

24. ABCD

The pudendal nerve leaves the pelvis through the greater sciatic foramen to enter the gluteal region. There it crosses beneath the ischial spine to enter Alcock's canal on the lateral wall of the ischio-rectal fossa where it divides into its three branches: the dorsal nerve of the clitoris, the inferior haemorrhoidal nerve and the perineal nerve.

25. BD

The inguinal ligament 'bridges over' two large muscles (the iliacus and psoas major), two vessels (the femoral artery and vein), and two nerves (the lateral cutaneous nerve of the thigh and the femoral nerve between the iliacus and psoas).

26. AC

The superficial inguinal ring lies just above the pubic tubercle. It is triangular in shape and has a base (medial half of pubic crest), an apex (directed upwards and laterally) and two crura (superior and inferior). As the spermatic cord passes through the ring, a thin sheath of fascia arises from the margins of the ring and surrounds the cord as the external spermatic fascia. This fascia, therefore, does not pass through the ring.

27. BCD

The conjoint tendon is formed of the tendinous lower fibres of the internal oblique and transversus aponeuroses. As these two muscles lie behind the external oblique, the conjoint tendon also lies behind the external oblique and the structures derived from it (inguinal and lacunar ligaments).

28. ABDE

The cremaster muscle is formed of fibres from the transversus and internal oblique muscles. As the round ligament (spermatic cord in the male) passes under the curved lower border of these muscles, it becomes surrounded by a series of loops of fibres which form the cremaster muscle. These fibres spiral around the round ligament and are attached to the pubic tubercle and the medial half of the inguinal ligament.

29. ABCE

Each adrenal gland rests on its corresponding crus of the diaphragm. The medial border of each gland is related to the coeliac ganglion on its side. Anteriorly, the right adrenal is related to the bare area of the liver laterally and the inferior vena cava medially. The lower pole of the left gland is covered in front by the tail of the pancreas. The rest of the gland is covered with peritoneum of the omental bursa and forms part of the bed of the stomach.

30. BCD

The inferior mesenteric artery is the artery of the hindgut. It arises from the front of the aorta at the inferior border of the third part of the duodenum, opposite the third lumbar vertebra. It gives off the upper left colic artery, the lower left colic artery and the sigmoid arteries. Over the pelvic brim, opposite the middle of the left common iliac artery it continues as the superior rectal artery.

31. ABD

The fascia transversalis lies behind the muscles of the anterior abdominal wall and in front of the parietal peritoneum. Above, it is continuous with the diaphragmatic fascia. At the inner lip of the iliac crest and the lateral half of the inguinal ligament it becomes continuous with the fascia iliaca; below that level the fascia transversalis forms the anterior wall of the femoral sheath while the fascia iliaca forms its posterior wall. Colles' fascia is the continuation of Scarpa's fascia in the perineum.

32. ADE

The ilio-inguinal nerve arises from the anterior primary ramus of L1 and pierces the psoas major muscle to emerge from under cover of its lateral border. It then descends laterally on the quadratus lumborum and behind the kidney before piercing the transversus muscle and running forward between that muscle and the internal oblique. At the level of the anterior superior iliac spine it pierces the internal oblique and runs between it and the external oblique before emerging from the superficial inguinal ring to supply the skin of the external genitalia. The skin over the mons is supplied by the iliohypogastric nerve.

33. ABD

The major structures supporting the uterus are those attached to the cervix, hence the relative lack of mobility in the cervix in comparison to the uterine body. These supporting structures are the utero-sacral, the pubo-cervical and the cardinal ligaments. The levator ani muscles also support the uterus by forming a shelf which prevents the downward displacement (prolapse) of the pelvic organs.

34. ADE

The quadratus lumborum muscle arises from the transverse process of the fifth lumbar vertebra, the ilio-lumbar ligament and the adjoining 5 cm of the inner lip of the iliac crest. It then passes upwards to the transverse processes of upper four lumbar vertebrae and the medial half of the lower border of the twelfth rib. It is supplied by T12 and L1–4 and acts as a muscle of inspiration by fixing the last rib while the diaphragm is contracting during inspiration. Additionally it causes abduction (lateral flexion) of the lumbar vertebrae. There is no rotatory movement at the lumbar vertebrae.

35. BCD

The subcutaneous tissue of the scrotum contains no fat, but has a sheet of involuntary muscle fibres (dartos muscle) which are adherent to the skin and to the deep layer of the superficial fascia (Colles' fascia). The dartos muscle is supplied by sympathetic fibres which are carried in the perineal branch of S4, and acts to wrinkle the skin of the scrotum in cold weather.

36. BCD

The gubernaculum is a mass of mesoderm attached between the lower pole of gonad (testis or ovary) and the labio-scrotal swelling (scrotum or labium majus). It passes through the inguinal canal and precedes the testis during its descent in intrauterine life. In the female it forms the ovarian and the round ligaments.

37. C

The inguinal canal lies parallel to and above the medial half of the inguinal ligament. It starts at the deep inguinal ring which lies lateral to the deep epigastric artery and ends at the superficial ring. Its posterior wall is formed by the transversalis fascia laterally and the conjoint tendon medially. Its anterior wall is formed by the external oblique aponeurosis, assisted laterally by the internal oblique muscle. The roof is formed by the lower edges of the internal oblique and the transversus abdominis muscles, and the floor by the grooved inner surface of the inguinal ligament, reinforced medially by the lacunar ligament.

38. CDE

The anatomy of the inguinal canal is the key to the understanding of inguinal hernias (*see question 37*). An oblique (indirect) hernia passes through the deep ring along the canal, hence A, B and C in the question are false for direct hernia but would have been true for indirect hernia. A direct hernia pushes its way directly forward (hence the name) through the posterior wall of the inguinal canal. Both types can leave the canal by passing through the superficial ring.

39. CDE

The femoral vessels, passing behind the inguinal ligament into the thigh, draw around themselves a prolongation of the fascia transversalis anteriorly and the fascia iliaca posteriorly to form the femoral sheath. These fasciae fuse with the adventitia of the vessels one inch below the inguinal ligament. They also fuse with the inguinal ligament lateral to the femoral artery, hence the femoral nerve enters the thigh outside the femoral sheath.

40. ACD

The coverings of the spermatic cord are the *internal spermatic fascia* (derived from the fascia transversalis at the deep ring), the *cremaster muscle and fascia* (derived from the internal oblique as the cord passes through the inguinal canal) and the *external spermatic fascia* (derived from the aponeurosis of the external oblique at the superficial ring). They are supplied by the cremasteric nerve (L2) and the ilio-inguinal nerve (L1). Their arterial supply is from the cremasteric artery, a branch of the inferior epigastric artery, while the arterial supply of the vas is from the artery to the vas, a branch of the inferior vesical artery.

41. ACDE

The vas deferens carries the sperm from the testis to the prostatic urethra. It starts behind the testis as a continuation of the canal of the epididymis and ends in a dilatation called the ampulla medial to the seminal vesicle. The ampulla joins the duct of the seminal vesicle to form the ejaculatory duct which opens into the prostatic urethra.

42. ACE

The abdominal organs (e.g. kidney) as well as those organs which developed embryologically in the abdomen (e.g. epididymis and testis) drain into the para-aortic lymph nodes.

43. BCE

During development the mesonephros is replaced by the metanephros and disappears except for some of its tubules which persist and form the vasa efferentia which drains the testis into the epididymis. Other mesonephric tubules persist in the male as remnants without serving any function. These include the appendix of the epididymis, the ductulus aberrans superior, the ductulus aberrans inferior, and the paradidymis. The appendix testis and the utriculus masculinus are remnants of the paramesonephric duct in the male.

44. ACE

The falciform ligament is formed of two leaves of the peritoneum connecting the liver to the diaphragm and the anterior abdominal wall. It is attached to the upper surface of the liver to the right of the midline (as the ligament is wide), to the central tendon of the diaphragm, and to the anterior abdominal wall along the linea alba from the xiphi-sternum to the umbilicus. Its free lower edge contains the ligamentum teres of the liver.

45. ACE

The epiploic foramen (the foramen of Winslow) connects the lesser sac to the greater sac and lies behind the free border of the lesser omentum. This free border contains the bile duct (in front and to the right), the hepatic artery (in front and to the left) and the portal vein (behind). Other boundaries of the foramen are: the inferior vena cava posteriorly, the first part of the duodenum inferiorly, and the caudate process of the liver superiorly.

46. ABE

The bare area of the liver lies on the right end of its posterior surface. It is triangular in shape; its base is the inferior vena cava, its upper and lower sides are the separated layers of the coronary ligament, and its apex is the right triangular ligament where these two layers meet. The bare area is in direct contact with the diaphragm, the inferior vena cava and the right adrenal gland.

47. BCE

Structures related to the posterior surface of the stomach are usually known as the stomach 'bed'. From below upwards they are: the transverse colon, the transverse mesocolon, the body of the pancreas, the splenic artery, the upper part of the left kidney, the left adrenal gland, the spleen and the left crus of the diaphragm.

48. ACD

The thyroid gland develops from the caudal end of the thyroglossal duct. It lies within the pretracheal fascia, to which it is not adherent except between the isthmus and the 2nd, 3rd and 4th tracheal rings.

49. BC

The recurrent laryngeal nerve lies deep to the pretracheal fascia, while the omo-hyoid muscle lies superficial to it. The main trunk of the inferior thyroid artery divides outside the pretracheal fascia into four or five branches which pierce the fascia to reach the lower pole of the thyroid gland. The superior thyroid artery, on the other hand, pierces the fascia as a single trunk before dividing into anterior and posterior branches.

50. ABCE

The internal anal sphincter is the thickened lower end of the inner circular muscle of the rectum. It is under voluntary control similar to the smooth muscle of the bladder. The internal sphincter is rather weak, and is not capable of maintaining continence when acting alone without the help of the external sphincter.

51. ADE

The anal canal is divided into an upper two-thirds (cloacal part) and a lower third (anal-pit part). The junction between these two parts is the Hilton's white line. The upper part is endodermal in origin, is lined with mucous membrane, has autonomic supply from the inferior hypogastric plexuses, drains its venous blood via the superior rectal vein to the portal system and drains its lymph to the lumbar lymph nodes. The lower part, on the other hand, is ectodermal in origin, is lined with thin hairless skin, has somatic supply from the inferior rectal nerve, drains its venous blood via inferior rectal vein to the systemic venous system and drains its lymph to the medial group of the superficial inguinal lymph nodes. Hilton's white line is avascular (hence the name), and there are no arterial or venous communications between the parts of the anal canal above and below it.

52. CDE

The superior rectal artery is the direct continuation of the inferior mesenteric artery (the artery of the hindgut). It touches, but does not cross, the medial side of the left ureter. There is very little anastomosis between the superior and the inferior rectal arteries.

53. BCE

The superior mesenteric artery arises from the front of the abdominal aorta at the level of the lower border of the body of L1. Its origin lies behind the neck of the pancreas and as it descends it passes in front of the following structures (in order): left renal vein, uncinate process of the pancreas, third part of duodenum, aorta, inferior vena cava, right psoas major muscle, right ureter, right ovarian (testicular) vessels and right genito-femoral nerve.

54. ABCD

The muscles lying in the floor of the femoral triangle are the iliacus, psoas major, pectineus, part of the adductor brevis and adductor longus.

55. BCE

The renal cortex contains the glomeruli and convoluted tubules, while the medulla contains the collecting tubules and the loop of Henle. Although the kidney is described as a 'retroperitoneal' organ, its anterior surface is not completely covered by peritoneum. Some structures lying on the kidney are also retroperitoneal and, thus, lift the peritoneum from its anterior surface. These structures are the right adrenal gland, right colic flexure and second part of duodenum (on the right kidney) and the left adrenal gland, descending colon and pancreas (on the left kidney). An abnormal renal artery passing behind the lower part of the renal pelvis might obstruct the ureter (which is the most posterior structure in the hilum) and cause hydronephrosis.

56. AC

The lesser sciatic foramen lies between the lesser sciatic notch and the sacrospinous and sacrotuberous ligaments. It transmits the tendon of obturator internus, nerve to obturator internus, internal pudendal vessels and pudendal nerve.

57. AE

The ureter is mesodermal in origin. It arises from the renal hilum behind the renal artery (which is behind the renal vein). It then descends on the medial edge of the psoas major which separates it from the tips of the transverse processes of the lumbar vertebrae (L2–L5). It receives blood supply from the aorta, renal, gonadal, common iliac, superior vesical and inferior vesical arteries.

58. BCE

The right ureter lies in front of the genito-femoral nerve and the ischial spine.

59. BDE

The trigone is relatively indistensible and immobile as compared with the fundus of the bladder. It overlies the median lobe of the prostate in the male and the uterine cervix and the anterior vaginal fornix in the female. The transitional epithelium of the bladder has no glands.

60. ABD

The urinary bladder is supplied by both sympathetic and parasympathetic fibres. The sympathetic fibres come from the hypogastric nerves and are inhibitory to the detrusor muscle and motor to the internal sphincter. The parasympathetic supply is via the pelvic plexus from the nervi erigentes and conveys pain and distension sensations. The lateral ligaments of the bladder are thickenings of the areolar tissue passing from the base of the bladder laterally across the pelvic floor.

61. ADE

The male urethra is formed of three parts: prostatic, membranous and penile. The *prostatic* part has a longitudinal ridge along its posterior wall called the urethral crest. In the middle of the urethral crest there is a rounded elevation called the seminal colliculus. On the summit of the seminal colliculus there is the opening of a small diverticulum called the prostatic utricle (analogous to the uterus in the female). The ejaculatory ducts open on the margins of the prostatic utricle. The gutter on either side of the urethral crest is called the prostatic sinus, where the prostatic ducts open. The *membranous* urethra lies in the deep perineal pouch. On either side lie the bulbo-urethral glands. Their ducts, however, pierce the perineal membrane to open into the *penile* urethra.

62. BCDE

The isthmus is the constricted area (0.5 cm wide) which lies between the uterine body and the cervix. The constriction at the upper end of the isthmus is the *anatomical internal os* which is marked externally by the reflection of the utero-vesical peritoneum. At the lower end of the isthmus lies the *histological internal* os where the endometrium changes into columnar cervical epithelium.

63. ABCDE

The main lymphatics of the uterus pass to the internal iliac lymph nodes. Some lymphatics from the fundus, however, pass along the round ligament to the superficial inguinal nodes.

64. AD

The ovary develops embryologically in the abdomen and, therefore, the ovarian artery arises from the aorta and the ovarian lymphatics drain into the para-aortic lymph nodes. It has no peritoneal coat and is covered with cubical epithelium known as the germinal epithelium.

65. ACD

The ovarian ligament is a fibromuscular cord connecting the lower pole of the ovary to the cornu of the uterus. It is covered by a fold of peritoneum (broad ligament). The ovarian vessels are contained in the infundibulo-pelvic ligament. Despite being attached to these two ligaments and to the mesovarium, the ovary is very mobile and has a variable position.

66. ABCD

The Fallopian tube develops from the para-mesonephric duct, while the ovary develops from the genital ridge.

67. CE

The vaginal portion of the cervix enters the vagina through its anterior wall, hence the posterior wall is 1–2 cm longer. There is no peritoneal covering over the anterior wall. There are no glands in the vagina; the lumen is kept moist by mucus secreted from the cervical glands.

68. ABCD

The paroöphoron and epoöphoron are vestigial remnants of the Wolffian ducts. The ovary is not covered with peritoneum and is not included in the broad ligament (which is a peritoneal fold).

69. B

The obturator nerve arises from the *ventral* primary rami of L2, 3 and 4 as part of the lumbar plexus in the substance of the psoas major muscle. It reaches the thigh by passing through the obturator canal. It provides muscular branches to the gracilis, obturator externus and the adductors of the thigh (longus, brevis and magnus).

It also provides articular branches to the hip and knee joints and cutaneous branches to the skin over the medial aspect of the thigh. The obturator internus muscle is supplied by a branch from the sacral plexus.

70. BD

The lumbar plexus is formed by the ventral primary rami of the upper four lumbar nerves in the substance of the psoas major muscle. The branches of this plexus emerge from the muscle as follows: the genito-femoral nerve through its anterior surface; the obturator nerve and lumbo-sacral trunk through its medial border; and the ilio-inguinal, ilio-hypogastric, femoral and lateral cutaneous nerve of the thigh through its lateral border. The sciatic nerve is a branch of the sacral plexus.

71. CDE

The female pelvis is shorter and wider than the male pelvis to accommodate its obstetric function. The sacro-iliac joint extends only to the lower border of the second piece of the sacrum. The greater sciatic notch is almost at a right-angle. In the upright position the following structures are at the same horizontal plane: upper border of the symphysis pubis, tip of the coccyx, ischial spine, centre of acetabulum, femoral head and tip of greater trochanter.

72. BCDE

The symphysis pubis (as the name implies) is a *secondary* cartilaginous joint. A primary cartilaginous joint is one where bone and hyaline cartilage meet, such as the junction of a rib with its costal cartilage. A secondary cartilaginous joint, on the other hand, is a union between bones whose articular surfaces are covered with thin lamina of hyaline cartilage. These laminae are united by fibro-cartilage.

73. BCE

The levator ani muscle originates from the posterior surface of the lower border of the body of the pubis, the ischial spine and the intervening white line on the obturator fascia. Despite its name, the ilio-coccygeus part does not arise from the ilium; the name derives from its former origin on the iliac bone at the pelvic brim, which is its origin in most mammals.

74. BDE

The internal iliac artery divides into an anterior and a posterior division. Branches of the anterior division are the umbilical (superior vesical), obturator, middle rectal, vaginal, uterine, inferior vesical, inferior gluteal and internal pudendal arteries. Branches of the posterior division are the ilio-lumbar, lateral sacral and superior gluteal arteries. The median sacral artery is a branch of the aorta and the superior rectal artery is the terminal branch of the inferior mesenteric artery.

75. AE

The great saphenous vein ascends in front of the medial malleolus where it lies immediately behind the saphenous nerve. The small saphenous vein drains into the popliteal vein.

76. ABE

The obturator artery gives off a pubic branch which anastomoses with the pubic branch of the inferior epigastric artery. In about 25–30% of people the obturator artery does not arise from the internal iliac and, in such cases, the pubic branch of the inferior epigastric becomes large enough to replace the obturator artery itself and is called the *abnormal obturator artery*.

77. ACD

The ischio-rectal fossa contains the inferior rectal nerve and vessels, the labial (scrotal) nerve and vessels, the perineal branch of the fourth sacral nerve and fat. The pudendal nerve and the internal pudendal artery are enclosed in the pudendal (Alcock's) canal which forms part of the lateral wall of the ischio-rectal fossa.

78. ABCE

The superficial perineal pouch lies between the perineal membrane and the superficial (Colles') fascia. In the female it contains the crus of the clitoris, the bulbs of the vestibule, the Bartholin's glands and the three superficial muscles: the ischio-cavernosus, the bulbo-spongiosus and the superficial transverse perinei.

79. CDE

The branches of the sacral plexus are the pudendal, sciatic, pelvic splanchnic, perforating cutaneous and the superior and inferior gluteal nerves. It also gives the posterior cutaneous nerve of the thigh as well as nerves to the obturator internus, quadratus femoris and piriformis muscles. The femoral nerve and the lateral cutaneous nerve of the thigh are branches of the lumbar plexus.

80. ACD

The diaphragmatic peritoneum is supplied centrally by the phrenic nerve and peripherally by the intercostal nerves. During expiration (whether forced or tranquil) the diaphragm is wholly passive.

6

Embryology and Genetics

81. Homologous structures in the male and the female are:

    A. the scrotum and the ovary.

    B. the bulbo-urethral (Cowper's) gland and the great vestibular (Bartholin's) gland.

    C. the penile urethra and the labia minora.

    D. the gubernaculum testis and the infundibulo-pelvic ligament of the ovary.

    E. the prostate and the para-urethra (Skene's) glands.

82. The mesonephric (Wolffian) duct:

    A. is present in the female embryo.

    B. forms the processus vaginalis.

    C. forms the epoöphoron.

    D. forms the testis.

    E. does not respond to testosterone unless it is converted to dihydrotestosterone.

83. The human oocyte:

    A. at ovulation is smaller than the human sperm.

    B. commences its first meiotic division at the age of puberty.

    C. contains a haploid number of chromosomes as a secondary oocyte.

    D. is connected to the surrounding granulosa cells by microvilli.

    E. develops from the germinal epithelium of the ovary.

84. The urogenital ridge gives rise to:
  A. the urinary bladder.
  B. the Fallopian tube.
  C. the ureter.
  D. the cervix.
  E. the vulva.

85. During embryological development:
  A. there are four umbilical vessels.
  B. the inferior parathyroid gland develops from the third pharyngeal pouch.
  C. the adrenal cortex and medulla develop from the mesoderm.
  D. the physiological umbilical hernia is reduced by the end of the tenth intrauterine week.
  E. the caudal end of the neural tube closes earlier than the cranial end.

86. Structures developing from the mesoderm include:
  A. the spleen.
  B. the liver.
  C. the heart.
  D. the serous membranes.
  E. the lens of the eye.

87. Regarding spermatogenesis in the human:
  A. the whole process takes about 70 to 80 days.
  B. spermatogonia divide by meiosis.
  C. the sperm move actively along the seminiferous tubules.
  D. one spermatogonium gives rise to four spermatids.
  E. the mid-piece of the mature sperm is rich in mitochondria.

88. An abnormal karyotype is a feature of:
  A. androgen insensitivity (testicular feminization) syndrome.
  B. Klinefelter's syndrome.
  C. Edward's syndrome.

   D. Marfan's syndrome.

   E. cystic fibrosis.

89. Conditions with autosomal dominant inheritance include:

   A. galactosaemia.

   B. multiple neurofibromatosis.

   C. haemophilia.

   D. tuberose sclerosis.

   E. osteogenesis imperfecta.

90. Nuclear chromatin (Barr body):

   A. represents an inactivated X chromosome which could be of paternal origin.

   B. is present in individuals with androgen insensitivity syndrome.

   C. is observed during interphase.

   D. does not appear in the cells of the normal female embryo until the ovaries have developed.

   E. is present in female Down's syndrome (trisomy 21).

91. In early human development:

   A. fertilization normally occurs in the ampullary part of the Fallopian tube.

   B. implantation occurs 2–3 days post-fertilization.

   C. implantation occurs at the stage of blastocyst.

   D. the second meiotic division of the sperm is completed after fertilization.

   E. the yolk sac develops within the inner cell mass.

92. Regarding Turner's syndrome (45,X):

   A. there is only one nuclear chromatin (Barr body).

   B. there is increased risk of spontaneous abortion in affected embryos.

   C. there is increased incidence with increased maternal age.

   D. no germ cells are present during intrauterine development.

   E. short stature is a phenotypic feature.

93. **The amniotic fluid:**

    A. is biochemically identical to fetal plasma during the first 20 weeks of pregnancy.

    B. exchanges fluid across the amnion covering the umbilical cord.

    C. has urea concentration which progressively decreases with increased gestation.

    D. has contribution from the fetal urine of about 500 ml per 24 hour at term.

    E. is usually reduced in volume in a fetus with anencephaly.

94. **During human development:**

    A. the thymus gland develops from the third pharyngeal pouch.

    B. the right fourth pharyngeal arch artery forms the arch of aorta.

    C. the spleen is a derivative of the foregut.

    D. the centre of the diaphragm develops from the septum transversum.

    E. the suprarenal medulla develops from the neural crest.

95. **In the fetal circulation:**

    A. the ductus arteriosus develops from the left sixth pharyngeal arch artery.

    B. the ductus venosus carries deoxygenated blood.

    C. there is high pulmonary vascular resistance.

    D. there is low placental vascular resistance.

    E. the pulmonary blood flow is about 25% of the cardiac output.

96. **Features of untreated Turner's syndrome (45,X) include:**

    A. low serum gonadotrophin levels.

    B. low serum oestrogen levels.

    C. hot flushes.

    D. lymphoedema.

    E. increased incidence of gonadal malignant tumours.

97. The amniotic fluid:

    A. is more alkaline than blood.

    B. has increased bilirubin concentration with increased gestation.

    C. contains glial cells in the presence of open neural tube defects.

    D. does not contain fibrinogen.

    E. has increased insulin concentration with increased gestation.

98. The vagina:

    A. develops partially from the urogenital sinus.

    B. recanalizes at 20 weeks post-conception.

    C. may be absent in the presence of ovaries.

    D. has a pH of 5 in the first few days of life.

    E. may be completely absent in the presence of a uterus.

99. In the development of the female genital system:

    A. the maximum number of oocytes is present at 20–22 weeks intrauterine life.

    B. the labia majora develop from the urogenital folds.

    C. the ovaries can be identified histologically at 7 weeks intrauterine life.

    D. by 12 weeks intrauterine life the external genitalia are distinct from those of the male.

    E. the ovaries have a mixed mesodermal and endodermal origin.

100. The placenta:

    A. develops from the decidua basalis and the chorion frondosum.

    B. is covered by the amnion on its fetal surface.

    C. weighs more than the fetus before 15 weeks gestation.

    D. is morphologically divided into 15–20 lobes on its fetal surface.

    E. has a decreased number of syncytial knots in diabetic pregnancies.

101. In human cytogenetics:

  A. the Y chromosome is acrocentric.

  B. trisomy 16 is the commonest trisomy found in first-trimester spontaneous abortions.

  C. trisomy 1 is present in almost 10% of first-trimester spontaneous abortions.

  D. a cause of trisomy is non-disjunction at meiosis.

  E. pentasomy of sex chromosomes is compatible with life.

102. An individual with the karyotype 46,XX t (X;7) (p21;q23) will have:

  A. a female phenotype.

  B. a normal number of chromosomes.

  C. a translocation involving the long arm of the X chromosome.

  D. a translocation involving band 7 of the X chromosome.

  E. increased risk of reproductive loss.

103. In meiosis:

  A. replication of the DNA occurs during the synthesis (S) phase of the second meiotic division.

  B. crossing over occurs during prophase of the first meiotic division.

  C. the X and Y chromosomes undergo end-to-end synapsis between their short arms.

  D. one primary oocyte gives rise to four ova.

  E. nondysjunction produces aneuploid gametes.

104. An individual with trisomy 21 (47,XX, +21):

  A. can produce chromosomally normal children.

  B. usually has an IQ of 25–50.

  C. has an increased incidence of Hirschsprung's disease.

  D. has an increased incidence of acute leukaemia.

  E. may result from chromosomal translocation.

105. The first meiotic division of the primary oocyte:

  A. may take up to 40 years to be completed.

  B. results in two secondary oocytes.

C. is completed after fertilization.

D. results in two cells with haploid number of chromosomes.

E. is always followed by the second meiotic division.

106. **In a balanced chromosomal reciprocal translocation carrier there is:**

A. normal number of chromosomes.

B. normal amount of genetic material.

C. normal arrangement of genetic material.

D. increased risk of reproductive loss.

E. greater risk of cytogenetically abnormal offspring if the carrier is a female rather than male.

107. **Aneuploidy include:**

A. Patau's syndrome.

B. Lesch-Nyhan syndrome.

C. Klinefelter's syndrome.

D. Peutz's syndrome.

E. Turner's syndrome.

108. **With regard to human sexual differentiation:**

A. the Müllerian inhibiting factor has a local action.

B. the presence of functioning testes will always lead to a male phenotype.

C. the testicular differentiation factor is present on the long arm of the Y chromosome.

D. the presence of functioning ovaries is necessary for the development of female phenotype.

E. oestrogen causes development of the Müllerian system.

109. **In human cytogenetics:**

A. deoxyribonucleic acid (DNA) is double-stranded.

B. material for DNA analysis in adults is usually obtained from erythrocytes.

C. the base adenine is always paired with thymine in DNA.

    D. alleles are non-identical genes occupying homologous loci in a pair of chromosomes.

    E. penetrance is the extent of gene expression.

110. **Autosomal recessive inheritance occurs in:**

    A. ABO blood groups.

    B. congenital adrenal hyperplasia.

    C. Friedreich's ataxia.

    D. vitamin D-resistant rickets.

    E. haemochromatosis.

▌ EMBRYOLOGY AND GENETICS: ANSWERS

81. BCE

The scrotum is homologous to the labium majus, while the testis is homologous to the ovary. The gubernaculum testis is the homologue of the ovarian ligament and the round ligament of the uterus.

82. AC

Both male and female embryos possess two pairs of genital ducts: the mesonephric (Wolffian) duct, which fully develops in the male but degenerates in the female, and the paramesonephric (Müllerian) duct, which fully develops in the female but degenerates in the male. The Wolffian duct can respond directly to testosterone, while the tissues of the external genitalia need testosterone to be converted first to dihydrotestosterone by the action of 5-alpha reductase. The processus vaginalis is a fold of peritoneum and the testis develops from the genital ridge.

83. CD

The oocyte develops from the primordial germ cells in the wall of the yolk sac, from where it migrates to the genital ridge. The primordial germ cells differentiate into oogonia by the twelfth week of intrauterine life and then develop into primary oocytes (diploid number of chromosomes). The primary oocyte undergoes the initial phase of the first meiotic division before birth. This division is arrested at the prophase stage and is resumed just prior to ovulation to produce a secondary oocyte (haploid number of chromosomes) and the first polar body. The secondary oocyte enters the second meiotic division, which is arrested at the metaphase and is only resumed after fertilization to produce a fertilized ovum and a second polar body. The first polar body may also divide into smaller polar bodies. The mature oocyte is 120 μm in diameter while the sperm is 60 μm long, the headpiece being only 5 μm in diameter.

84. BCD

All the organs of the genito-urinary system (with the exception of the bladder, urethra and vulva) develop from the urogenital ridge.

85. ABD

Originally there are two umbilical arteries and two umbilical veins in the embryo. As development proceeds, by about day 34 post-fertilization, the right umbilical vein degenerates while the left vein remains. The adrenal gland has a mixed origin: the cortex from the ectoderm and the medulla from the mesoderm. The cranial end of the neural tube closes earlier than the caudal end (at 24 and 26 days post-fertilization, respectively), hence neural tube defects are usually in the lumbo-sacral region.

86. ACD

The liver is endodermal in origin, while the lens is ectodermal.

87. ADE

Spermatogonia divide by mitosis to form primary spermatocytes which go through the first meiotic division to form secondary spermatocytes. These enter the second meiotic division to form spermatids, which are then transformed into mature spermatozoa by the process of spermiogenesis. Sperm are carried passively along the seminiferous tubules by the contraction of the surrounding muscle cells.

88. BC

Klinefelter's syndrome is 47,XXY and Edward's syndrome is trisomy 18.

89. BDE

Galactosaemia is autosomal recessive and haemophilia is X-linked recessive.

90. ACE

Nuclear chromatin (Barr body) represents an inactivated X chromosome, which may be maternal or paternal in origin. It appears early, probably around the time of implantation. During interphase the number of Barr bodies present in a nucleus is one less than the number of X chromosomes present. In androgen insensitivity syndrome (46,XY) there are no Barr bodies, while in female Down's (47,XX,+21) there is one.

91. ACE

Implantation takes place about 6 days after fertilization. The second meiotic division of the sperm is completed while it is still in the seminiferous tubules. On the other hand, the second meiotic division of the oocyte is not completed until after fertilization.

92. BE

As the number of Barr bodies present in a nucleus is one less than the number of X chromosomes present, there are no Barr bodies in Turner's syndrome. During early intrauterine development there is a normal number of germ cells. These germ cells, however, fail to surround themselves with granulosa cells during development, do not form follicles and are destroyed before term.

93. ABD

The amniotic fluid urea and creatinine levels increase progressively with increased gestation, reflecting increasing contribution from fetal urine. Anencephalic fetuses have impaired swallowing and hence increased liquor volume.

94. ADE

The right fourth pharyngeal arch artery forms the right subclavian artery, while the left fourth pharyngeal arch artery forms the arch of aorta. The spleen arises from cellular islands in the coelomic epithelium.

95. ACD

The ductus venosus carries oxygenated blood to the inferior vena cava. The pulmonary blood flow in the fetus is only 3–7% of the cardiac output.

96. BD

In Turner's syndrome there is hypergonadotrophic hypogonadism. Despite low oestrogen levels, these women do not have hot flushes. Only after oestrogen is administered and withdrawn do they experience hot flushes. The incidence of gonadal malignant tumours is increased only where there is a Y chromosome in the karyotype (e.g. mosaic 45X/46XY).

97. CDE

The amniotic fluid is slightly acidic (pH 7.0) when compared with blood. The bilirubin levels normally decrease with increasing gestational age except in cases of fetal haemolysis.

98. ABCDE

The vagina develops partially from the urogenital sinus and partially from the paramesonephric ducts. The uterus also develops from the paramesonephric duct. Therefore, in cases of congenital malformations, it would be expected that the presence of a uterus is associated with the presence of the upper part of the vagina at least. Nevertheless, malformations are by definition abnormal and there are many malformations which could not be explained by the normal development (such as item E in the question).

99. ADE

The labia minor and majora develop from the urogenital folds and swellings, respectively. The testes could be identified histologically at 7 weeks intrauterine life, but the ovaries not until 20 weeks.

100. ABC

The maternal surface of the placenta is divided into lobes, while the fetal surface is smooth. Syncytial knots represent segments of the syncytiotrophoblast in which the syncytial cell nuclei are packed together. They occur in the normal placenta and their number increases *in vivo* in diabetic pregnancies and *in vitro* if the villi from normal placentas are cultured under hypoxic conditions. They are thought to enhance placental transfer.

101. ABDE

Almost half of first-trimester spontaneous abortions are chromosomally abnormal. The majority of these abnormalities are trisomies (about 60%). Trisomies have been described for all chromosomes except number 1 and the Y chromosome. The commonest is trisomy 16 (about 32% of all trisomies).

102. ABE

There is an internationally agreed chromosomal nomenclature. The chromosomal complement is designated by: 1) the total number of chromosomes, 2) the sex chromosomal complement, and 3) any specific abnormality. 't' refers to translocation, 'del' to deletion, 'i' to isochromosome, and 'r' to ring chromosome. A karyotype containing additional or missing autosomes is signified by '+' and '−', respectively, followed by the number of the chromosome affected (e.g. female trisomy 21: 47, XX, +21). The chromosome having the lower number is recorded first, but if a sex chromosome is involved, this comes first. 'p' refers to the short arm while 'q' refers to the long arm. Numbers following 'p' or 'q' refer to the band affected. In the given example in the question the total number is 46 (normal), the sex chromosomes are XX (female phenotype). There is translocation between band 21 on the short arm of chromosome X and band 23 on the long arm of chromosome 7.

103. BCE

In the second meiotic division there is no DNA synthesis, this having occurred in the first meiotic division. During the first division also there is pairing (synapsis) between homologous chromosomes prior to exchange of genetic material (crossing over). Autosomes undergo side-to-side synapsis while the X and Y chromosomes undergo end-to-end synapsis between their short arms. One primary oocyte gives rise to one ovum and two polar bodies.

104. ABCD

Down's syndrome can result from chromosomal translocation, but the question specified trisomy 21, which results from non-dysjunction.

105. AD

The primary oocyte commences its first meiotic division *in utero*. This division is arrested during prophase and is only completed at ovulation (which may occur some 50 years later) to produce a secondary oocyte and a polar body. The secondary oocyte will undergo the second meiotic division only after fertilization.

106. ABDE

In translocation the chromosomes become broken (during meiosis or mitosis) and the resulting fragments become joined to other chromosomes. Reciprocal translocation involves an exchange of material between two non-homologous chromosomes. In balanced translocation there is a normal number of chromosomes and amount of genetic material but this material is rearranged. These individuals are phenotypically normal, but have increased risk of producing offsprings with abnormal amounts of genetic material (unbalanced translocation).

107. ACE

Aneuploidy is any deviation from the normal 46 chromosomes. It includes Patau's syndrome (trisomy 13), Klinefelter's syndrome

(47, XXY), and Turner's syndrome (45, X). In Peutz's syndrome (multiple polyposis of the intestines) and Lesch-Nyhan syndrome there are no recognizable chromosomal abnormalities.

108. AC

Sexual differentiation depends on the sex chromosomes, gonadal differentiation and end organ's response. In the presence of a Y chromosome (in addition to at least one X) the indifferent gonads will become testes. The absence of a Y chromosome (in the presence of at least one X) will lead to gonadal differentiation as ovaries. The testes will produce testosterone and Müllerian inhibitor. Testosterone will cause development of the male (Wolffian) duct system by direct action. The external genitalia, however, cannot respond to testosterone directly, but need it to be converted to dihydrotestosterone by action of the enzyme 5-alpha reductase. In cases of 5-alpha reductase deficiency there will be functioning testes but female phenotype. The Müllerian inhibitor causes regression of the female (Müllerian) duct system. In the female it is the absence of testes, and hence testosterone and Müllerian inhibitor, that leads to female phenotype and the development of the Müllerian system.

109. ACDE

Erythrocytes are anucleated and therefore are not used for DNA analysis. DNA is usually obtained from leukocytes.

110. BCE

The mode of inheritance in ABO blood groups is codominant (both alleles are expressed fully and equally) and in vitamin D-resistant rickets is X-linked dominant.

7

Maternal and Fetal Physiology

111. Alpha-fetoprotein:

   A. is a glycoprotein.

   B. is produced in the yolk sac.

   C. reaches its highest concentration in the maternal serum at about 16 weeks gestation.

   D. has similar concentration in the fetal serum and the amniotic fluid.

   E. has abnormally reduced concentration in second trimester maternal serum in cases of Down's syndrome (47, +21).

112. Human chorionic gonadotrophin:

   A. is a glycoprotein.

   B. is secreted by the syncytiotrophoblasts.

   C. reaches its maximal concentration in maternal serum at 36 to 38 weeks gestation.

   D. may be detected in the maternal blood before the expected date of the missed period, i.e. prior to 14 days post-fertilization.

   E. may be detected in maternal blood at 7 days after first-trimester abortion.

113. The following statements are correct:

   A. one millimole of an ion is the molecular weight in milligrams.

   B. one millimole is equal to 1 mole $\times 10^{-6}$.

   C. one milliequivalent (mEq) of sodium is equal to 1 millimole.

    D. a physiological solution of sodium chloride (0.9%) contains a sodium concentration of 9 millimole/litre.

    E. sodium is the principal cation in interstitial fluid.

114. Plasma:

    A. increases in volume during pregnancy in proportion to the size of the fetus.

    B. contains relatively less protein than the interstitial fluid.

    C. contains relatively more sodium than the interstitial fluid.

    D. has chloride as its major anion.

    E. has potassium as its major cation.

115. The anion gap is increased in:

    A. hypercalcaemia.

    B. methanol poisoning.

    C. hyperchloraemic acidosis.

    D. diabetic ketoacidosis.

    E. salicylate poisoning.

116. The osmotic pressure of the plasma:

    A. is decreased during pregnancy.

    B. is mainly due to its protein content.

    C. at the arteriolar end of the capillary causes passage of water into the interstitial space.

    D. when increased leads to increased secretion of vasopressin.

    E. is higher in the renal glomerular capillaries than that in other capillaries.

117. The following substances are paired with the mechanism of their placental transfer:

    A. oxygen–simple diffusion.

    B. carbohydrates–active transport.

    C. amino acids–facilitated diffusion.

    D. immunoglobulin M (IgM)–pinocytosis.

    E. fatty acids–simple diffusion.

118. The cerebrospinal fluid:

    A. is more acidic than plasma.

    B. has a volume of about 130–150 ml.

    C. has a normal pressure of 7–18 cm H_2O at the lumbar region.

    D. is produced at a rate of about 500 ml/day.

    E. has similar osmolality to plasma.

119. The pH (7.4) of plasma at normal body temperature:

    A. is neutral.

    B. represents hydrogen ion concentration of 0.00004 mmol/l.

    C. is more alkaline than the pH of the pancreatic juice.

    D. could be calculated using the Henderson–Hasselbalch equation.

    E. increases in metabolic acidosis.

120. Haemoglobin:

    A. has six times the buffering capacity of plasma proteins.

    B. is a weaker buffer in its deoxygenated form than in the oxygenated form.

    C. in its fetal form (Hb F) binds 2,3-diphosphoglycerate less effectively than adult haemoglobin (Hb A).

    D. decreases in concentration during normal pregnancy.

    E. is increased in its glycosylated form (Hb A_{1C}) in poorly controlled diabetes mellitus.

121. Metabolic acidosis:

    A. is associated with uretero-sigmoid anastomosis.

    B. may be caused by excessive vomiting.

    C. occurs in cardiac arrest.

    D. should be corrected with sodium bicarbonate in cases of renal failure.

    E. may occur in neonatal respiratory distress syndrome.

122. Changes associated with normal pregnancy include:

    A. increased red cell fragility.

    B. hyperventilation.

    C. respiratory alkalosis.

    D. increased levels of alkaline phosphatase.

    E. decreased levels of aldosterone.

123. **In the human heart:**

    A. the electrical events of the electrocardiogram precede the mechanical events.

    B. there is a rise in atrial pressure during the isometric ventricular contraction phase.

    C. about 50 ml of blood remain in each ventricle at the end of systole.

    D. the ventricular ejection fraction at rest is 90%.

    E. during inspiration, the aortic valve closes slightly before the pulmonary valve.

124. **Pathological factors affecting fetal heart rate include:**

    A. maternal thyroid status.

    B. structural abnormalities of the fetal heart.

    C. maternal pyrexia.

    D. fetal sleep/activity state.

    E. fetal anaemia.

125. **The P–R interval in the electrocardiogram:**

    A. is measured from the beginning of the P wave to the beginning of the R wave.

    B. may be prolonged in cases of hypokalaemia.

    C. is normally between 0.1 and 0.2 seconds.

    D. represents the time in which atrial depolarization and conduction through the atrio-ventricular node occur.

    E. coincides with the **v** wave in the jugular venous pressure trace.

126. **Normal changes in the electrocardiogram during pregnancy include:**

    A. deviation of the electrical axis to the left.

    B. a loud third heart sound.

    C. Q wave in lead III.

   D. shortened P-R interval.

   E. increased rate.

127. **In the normal human heart:**

   A. the oxygen saturation of blood in the left atrium and blood in the left ventricle is similar.

   B. the pressure in the pulmonary artery should not exceed 35 mmHg.

   C. the pressure in the right ventricle is about 35 mmHg throughout the cardiac cycle.

   D. the pressure in the left ventricle is about 10 mmHg at the end of diastole.

   E. the pacemaker is the sinoatrial node.

128. **The Q–T interval in the electrocardiogram is:**

   A. the period during which ventricular depolarization and repolarization occur.

   B. truly prolonged in hypocalcaemia.

   C. truly prolonged in hypokalaemia.

   D. more dependent on the heart rate than is the P–R interval.

   E. normally 3–4 seconds.

129. **The second heart sound:**

   A. is due to the opening of the aortic and pulmonary valves.

   B. has a pulmonary component which precedes the aortic component.

   C. has wide splitting during deep inspiration.

   D. occurs during the protodiastolic phase of the cardiac cycle.

   E. at birth is normally single with no splitting.

130. **Factors affecting ventricular end-diastolic volume include:**

   A. physical exercise.

   B. stimulation of the sympathetic nerve supply to the heart.

   C. intrathoracic pressure.

   D. atrial contraction.

   E. standing position.

131. Myocardial contractility is reduced in:

    A. acidosis.

    B. hypercapnia.

    C. treatment with ritodrine.

    D. myocardial infarction.

    E. treatment with quinidine.

132. During normal pregnancy there is an increase in:

    A. cardiac output mainly due to increased heart rate.

    B. arteriovenous oxygen gradient.

    C. red cell mass.

    D. haematocrit.

    E. blood volume proportional to the size of the fetus.

133. Renin:

    A. is a glycoprotein.

    B. is produced by the pregnant uterus.

    C. converts angiotensin I to angiotensin II.

    D. is synthesized as prorenin.

    E. secretion is increased during pregnancy.

134. Angiotensin II:

    A. is a decapeptide.

    B. is mainly formed in the lungs.

    C. sensitivity is increased in normal pregnancy.

    D. is metabolized into angiotensin III which is biologically inactive.

    E. stimulates aldosterone secretion.

135. During the second trimester of pregnancy there is normally an increase in:

    A. pulmonary capillary wedge pressure.

    B. central venous pressure.

    C. pulmonary blood flow.

    D. pulmonary arterial pressure.

    E. pulmonary vascular resistance.

136. During intrauterine life:

    A. the male fetus grows at a higher rate than the female fetus from the 24th week of gestation.

    B. the placenta grows at a slower rate than the fetus during the third trimester.

    C. the lungs are not capable of exchanging gases sufficient to support life before the 28th week of gestation.

    D. the fetal blood glucose levels are higher than those of the mother.

    E. fetal arterial pressure increases throughout pregnancy.

137. Brown fat cells (adipocytes):

    A. are innervated with sympathetic nerve fibres.

    B. each contains a single droplet of fat.

    C. contain mitochondria.

    D. are the major site of fat storage in the fetus.

    E. when stimulated they enhance heat production through shivering.

138. During normal pregnancy there is a fall in the serum levels of:

    A. sodium.

    B. potassium.

    C. calcium.

    D. magnesium.

    E. copper.

139. A positive Kleihauer test may be found:

    A. during the neonatal period.

    B. in men with sickle cell anaemia.

    C. in women with homozygous beta-thalassaemia.

    D. following feto-maternal haemorrhage.

    E. following normal delivery.

140. Alveolar air in the lungs:

    A. is fully saturated with water.

    B. has lower partial pressure of oxygen (PO_2) than expired air.

    C. is virtually totally replaced with every inspiration.

    D. has higher partial pressure of carbon dioxide (PCO_2) than expired air.

    E. is about 0.5 litre in total volume at the end of expiration.

141. The total respiratory dead space volume:

    A. has almost equal anatomical and alveolar components in a healthy resting individual.

    B. is usually one-third of the tidal volume.

    C. is reduced by breathing through a respiratory valve.

    D. is increased in an individual with pulmonary embolus.

    E. is increased in hyperventilation.

142. The functional residual capacity is:

    A. the volume of air in the lungs when the recoil of the chest wall and the recoil of the lungs are equal and opposite.

    B. reduced during normal pregnancy.

    C. smaller in women than it is in men.

    D. the volume of air left in the lungs after a maximal expiratory effort.

    E. increased with age in adults.

143. During pregnancy there is an increase in:

    A. the respiratory rate.

    B. the tidal volume.

    C. the vital capacity.

    D. the inspiratory capacity.

    E. the total lung capacity.

144. Intrapleural pressure:

    A. may exceed atmospheric pressure at the end of forced expiration.

    B. is lower (i.e. less negative) at the lung bases than the lung apex in the upright position.

    C. is decreased in older people.

    D. is transmitted to the oesophagus.

    E. may be as low as minus 30 mmHg at the end of forced inspiration.

145. Lung surfactants:

    A. are produced by type I pneumocytes.

    B. production is accelerated by glucocorticoid hormones.

    C. help to prevent pulmonary oedema.

    D. contain up to 8% proteins.

    E. may be deficient in cases of adult respiratory distress syndrome.

146. During pregnancy:

    A. there is about 40% increase in ventilation.

    B. the affinity of maternal haemoglobin to oxygen is decreased.

    C. the threshold of the respiratory centre to CO_2 is increased.

    D. the peak expiratory flow rate is unchanged.

    E. the forced expiratory volume in one second (FEV_1) is increased.

147. The carotid body chemoreceptors are:

    A. innervated by the glossopharyngeal nerve.

    B. stimulated in cases of carbon monoxide poisoning.

    C. stimulated in cases of cyanide poisoning.

    D. more sensitive to changes in the oxygen content of the blood than to its partial pressure (PO_2).

    E. stimulated by a rise in the hydrogen ion concentration.

148. Hyperventilation may lead to:

    A. decreased cerebral blood flow.

    B. tetany.

    C. increased cardiac output.

    D. respiratory alkalosis.

    E. significant elevation in blood pressure.

149. The sensitivity of the respiratory centres to CO_2 is increased in:

A. old age.

B. trained athletes.

C. pregnancy.

D. hypoxia.

E. metabolic acidosis.

150. The concentration of 2,3-diphosphoglycerate (2,3-DPG) in the red blood cells is increased by:

A. physical exercise

B. the presence of fetal haemoglobin (Hb F).

C. living at high altitude.

D. acidosis.

E. androgens.

151. The affinity of haemoglobin for oxygen is decreased by an increase in:

A. blood pH.

B. temperature.

C. 2,3-diphosphoglycerate.

D. carboxyhaemoglobin.

E. haemoglobin S.

152. Carbon dioxide in blood is:

A. more soluble than oxygen.

B. carried in combination with plasma proteins.

C. hydrated mainly in the plasma.

D. carried mainly as bicarbonate.

E. transported mainly in the red cells.

153. Fetal haemoglobin:

A. in its pure form has a high affinity for oxygen.

B. is formed of two alpha-chains and two gamma-chains.

C. forms less than 10% of the total haemoglobin by 4 months of age.

   D. is about 1% of the total haemoglobin in a normal adult.

   E. is formed in the yolk sac.

154. Cyanosis can be caused by:

   A. pulmonary oedema.

   B. carbon monoxide poisoning.

   C. left to right cardiac shunts.

   D. a low ventilation/perfusion (V/Q) ratio in one lung only.

   E. histotoxic hypoxia.

155. In the human kidney:

   A. the reabsorption of ions and water occurs mainly in the distal convoluted tubules.

   B. the renal plasma flow is normally 1.2 litre/minute.

   C. the glomerular filtration rate is proportional to body surface area.

   D. the filtration fraction increases in hypotension.

   E. blood flow in the cortex is greater than that in the medulla.

156. Fetal urine:

   A. production is reduced in cases of intrauterine growth retardation.

   B. is the major contributor to the amniotic fluid volume in the third trimester.

   C. is hypertonic with respect to fetal plasma.

   D. production is increased with advanced gestation.

   E. production is reduced in all cases of oligohydramnios.

157. During pregnancy there is an increase in:

   A. kidney length.

   B. renal blood flow.

   C. the diameter of the ureters, more pronounced on the right side.

   D. blood urea concentration.

   E. plasma osmolality.

158. Normal urodynamic findings in the adult female:

    A. voiding pressure: 45–70 mmHg.

    B. residual urine: = 50 ml.

    C. first sensation of bladder filling: 150–200 ml.

    D. maximum voiding pressure: = 70 cm H_2O.

    E. bladder capacity: 400–600 ml.

159. In the proximal convoluted tubules there is active reabsorption of:

    A. potassium.

    B. chloride.

    C. glucose.

    D. amino acids.

    E. sodium.

160. In the human kidney sodium is actively reabsorbed in:

    A. the proximal convoluted tubules.

    B. the loop of Henle.

    C. the distal convoluted tubules.

    D. the collecting tubules.

    E. the urinary bladder.

161. Erythropoietin:

    A. is a lipoprotein.

    B. is produced mainly in the kidney during intrauterine life.

    C. is mainly inactivated in the liver.

    D. production increases at high altitudes.

    E. stimulates the formation of proerythrocytes from stem cells.

162. With regard to normal micturition in the adult female:

    A. the intravesical pressure rises significantly during bladder filling.

    B. the urethra empties by gravity after urination.

    C. the pubo-rectalis muscle relaxes before the detrusor muscle contracts.

D. the intravesical pressure rise during urination can be augmented voluntarily.

E. the sensation of bladder filling is conveyed via the pelvic splanchnic nerve.

163. During normal pregnancy there is an increase in:

A. gastric acid secretion.

B. stomach emptying time.

C. liver blood flow.

D. water reabsorption in the large intestine.

E. plasma protein concentration.

164. In the normal fetus:

A. intestinal peristaltic movements appear as early as 12 weeks gestation.

B. the life span of the fetal erythrocyte is shorter than that of the normal adult erythrocyte.

C. swallowing plays a role in regulating amniotic fluid volume in the third trimester.

D. glycogen storage in the liver decreases towards term.

E. the liver is relatively immature in its ability to conjugate free bilirubin.

165. The gastric acid secretion is increased in:

A. hypoglycaemia.

B. the presence of food in the mouth.

C. the presence of food in the stomach.

D. the presence of fats and carbohydrates in the duodenum.

E. Zollinger–Ellison syndrome.

166. Factors which increase gastrin secretion include:

A. glucagon.

B. calcitonin.

C. calcium.

D. vagal stimulation.

E. atropine.

167. The normal gastric secretion:

    A. has a pH of 2.5.

    B. is produced at a rate of about 2.5 litres per day.

    C. contains glycoprotein.

    D. has sodium ion concentration which is inversely proportional to its hydrogen ion concentration.

    E. contains water.

168. During normal pregnancy there is an increase in plasma concentration of:

    A. phospholipids.

    B. albumin.

    C. beta-globulin.

    D. alanine aminotransferase.

    E. gamma-globulin.

169. Calcium:

    A. plasma levels are decreased after the menopause.

    B. is about 45% bound to protein in the plasma.

    C. excretion in the kidney is increased by calcitonin.

    D. reabsorption from bone by osteoclasts is inhibited by 1,25-dihydroxycholecalciferol.

    E. deficiency can lead to tetany.

170. Fetal breathing movements:

    A. increase within 48 hours of the onset of labour.

    B. are associated with the passage of meconium.

    C. may be reduced in fetal hypoxia.

    D. are primarily due to the movements of the intercostal muscles.

    E. are associated with gaseous exchange within the lungs.

171. Regarding the innervation of the female lower urinary tract:

    A. afferent fibres from the bladder ascend in the lateral reticulospinal tract.

    B. the periurethral muscle is supplied by the pudendal nerve.

C. the external urethral sphincter (rhabdosphincter) is supplied via the pelvic splanchnic nerves.

D. pudendal nerve block causes incontinence.

E. the rhabdosphincter receives a somatic supply from sacral roots S2–4.

172. Rapid eye movement (REM) sleep is associated with:

A. high-amplitude slow-frequency electroencephalogram activity.

B. increased skeletal muscle tone.

C. increased threshold for arousal by sensory stimuli as compared with non-REM sleep.

D. nocturnal enuresis.

E. desynchronization of the electroencephalogram activity.

173. In a reflex arc connecting a sense organ to a muscle there is a graded response (that is proportional to the magnitude of the stimulus) at:

A. the afferent axon.

B. the neuromuscular junction.

C. the muscle membrane.

D. the synapse between the afferent and efferent neurons.

E. the efferent axon.

174. The nerve fibres of the lateral corticospinal tract:

A. are mainly responsible for the coordination of voluntary movements.

B. originate in the precentral gyrus of the brain.

C. completely cross the midline at the pyramidal decussation in the medulla.

D. carry inhibitory signals to the deep reflexes.

E. descend through the internal capsule of the brain.

175. Pain sensation is:

A. transmitted through the lateral spinothalamic tract.

B. transmitted exclusively through myelinated nerve fibres.

    C. transmitted through nerve fibres which are larger in diameter than motor nerve fibre.

    D. not perceived by individuals who have extensive damage to the sensory area in their cerebral cortex.

    E. carried by nerve fibres which synapse in the substantia gelatinosa before crossing to the opposite side of the spinal cord.

176. **In the autonomic nervous system:**

    A. all the efferent thoracic preganglionic sympathetic nerves synapse in the paravertebral ganglion chain.

    B. the parasympathetic outflow to the head is via the III, VII and IX cranial nerves.

    C. the preganglionic sympathetic fibres supplying the uterus synapse in the inferior mesenteric ganglion.

    D. the adrenal medulla is innervated by relatively short post-ganglionic sympathetic fibres.

    E. the parasympathetic supply to the female external genitalia is via the pelvic nerve (sacral nerves 2, 3 and 4).

177. **Acetylcholine is the chemical transmitter at:**

    A. the sympathetic ganglion.

    B. the parasympathetic ganglion.

    C. the end of the postganglionic parasympathetic fibres.

    D. the end of the postganglionic sympathetic fibres to the pulmonary blood vessels.

    E. the end of the postganglionic sympathetic fibres to the sweat glands.

178. **Cholinergic stimulation causes contraction of:**

    A. the radial muscle of the iris.

    B. the ciliary muscles of the eye.

    C. the detrusor muscle of the bladder.

    D. the muscles in the trigone of the bladder.

    E. the bronchial muscles.

179. **Stimulation of catecholamine beta-2 receptors in:**

    A. the pregnant uterus causes decreased contraction.

    B. the systemic veins causes vasodilatation.

    C. the juxtaglomerular cells causes increased renin secretion.

    D. the spleen causes contraction of its capsule.

    E. the renal arterioles causes dilatation.

180. **Catecholamine beta-2 receptors are stimulated by:**

    A. adrenaline.

    B. noradrenaline.

    C. propranolol.

    D. ritodrine.

    E. metaraminol.

181. **Iron absorption from the gastrointestinal tract is inhibited by:**

    A. ascorbic acid.

    B. phosphates.

    C. phytates.

    D. gastric secretion.

    E. pancreatic secretion.

182. **Ferritin:**

    A. is a glycoprotein.

    B. represents 50% of the total body iron.

    C. is the main form of stored iron in the body.

    D. concentration in the umbilical cord blood is greater than that in the maternal blood.

    E. concentration is affected by recent ingestion of iron.

183. **Iron:**

    A. absorption occurs mainly in the duodenum.

    B. deficiency anaemia is frequent after partial gastrectomy.

    C. is stored in the body in the macrophages of the reticuloendothelial system.

D.   is transferred across the placenta by active transport.

E.   absorption is increased in pregnancy.

184. Iron deficiency anaemia in pregnancy is associated with a reduction in:

A.   mean red cell volume.

B.   serum iron concentration.

C.   total iron binding capacity.

D.   haemoglobin concentration.

E.   mean red cell haemoglobin.

185. Prostacyclin:

A.   is synthesized by platelets.

B.   promotes vasoconstriction.

C.   has a half-life of 30 minutes at body temperature.

D.   synthesis is inhibited by aspirin.

E.   is derived from arachidonic acid through the cyclo-oxygenase pathway.

186. Platelets:

A.   produce thromboxane A_2.

B.   have a half-life of about 4 days.

C.   count is reduced after splenectomy.

D.   count is reduced in severe pre-eclampsia.

E.   life-span is shortened in pre-eclampsia.

187. Lymph:

A.   fluid clots on standing at room temperature.

B.   fluid contains protein at a higher concentration than that of plasma.

C.   vessels contain valves.

D.   flow is mainly due to the contraction of skeletal muscles.

E.   flow is normally 2–4 litres/24 hours.

188. During pregnancy there is an increase in:

    A. clotting factor X concentration.

    B. fibrinolytic activity.

    C. antithrombin III concentration.

    D. fibrinogen concentration.

    E. erythrocyte sedimentation rate.

189. Tissue plasminogen activators:

    A. increase in concentration after surgical trauma.

    B. are abundant in the human placental tissue.

    C. have greater activity in veins than they have in arteries.

    D. are stimulated by tranexamic acid.

    E. are abundant in the ovarian tissue.

190. Compared with the adult, the neonate has reduced concentration of:

    A. vitamin K.

    B. protein S.

    C. clotting factor VIII.

    D. antithrombin III.

    E. clotting factor X.

▌MATERNAL AND FETAL PHYSIOLOGY: ANSWERS

111. ABE

Alpha-fetoprotein (AFP) is produced in the yolk sac, fetal liver and fetal gastrointestinal tract. Concentration in fetal serum rises from the fourth week of gestation to peak at 12–14 weeks and then progressively falls towards term. Amniotic fluid AFP concentration runs parallel to fetal serum concentration but is approximately 150 times lower. Maternal serum AFP concentration is approximately 50 000 times lower and lags behind that in the fetus, rising from weeks 10 to 32 and declining thereafter.

112. ABDE

Human chorionic gonadotrophin (hCG) can be detected in maternal serum as early as 7–9 days after fertilization. Initially, hCG concentration increases rapidly, doubling roughly every 48 hours. It reaches a peak at 8–10 weeks gestation before falling to plateau from about 20 weeks until term. With the current sensitive radioimmunoassays, hCG may be detected up to three weeks following delivery or abortion.

113. ACE

One millimole is equal to 1 mole $\times 10^{-3}$, while one micromole is equal to 1 mole $\times 10^{-6}$. A physiological solution of sodium chloride (0.9%) contains sodium concentration equal to the total number of cations in plasma (154 mmol/litre).

114. ACD

Plasma contains relatively more protein and sodium than the interstitial fluid. The major cation in plasma (and other extracellular fluids) is sodium, while potassium and, to a lesser extent, magnesium, are the principal cations in intracellular fluid.

115. BDE

The anion gap is the difference between the concentration of cations other than sodium and the concentration of anions other than chloride and bicarbonate in the plasma. Its normal range is 8–16 mEq/litre and is increased when organic acids or anions are increased or when plasma concentration of cations (potassium, calcium or magnesium ions) is decreased. It is decreased when cations are increased or when plasma albumin is decreased. It is not increased in hyperchloraemic acidosis.

116. ADE

The principal osmotic component of the plasma is sodium together with its accompanying anions, particularly chloride and bicarbonate, contributing about 270 mosmol/litre. The plasma proteins contribute less than 2 mosmol/litre because of their large molecular weights. At the arteriolar end of the capillary water passes into the interstitial space because of the hydrostatic pressure and not the osmotic pressure.

117. AE

Carbohydrates cross the placenta by facilitated diffusion and amino acids by active transport. IgM does not cross the placenta but IgG does, by the process of pinocytosis.

118. ABDE

The cerebrospinal fluid (CSF) fills the cerebral ventricles and the subarachnoid space. It is alkaline, but more acidic than plasma (CSF pH 7.33, plasma pH 7.40). It has a lumbar pressure of 7–18 cm of CSF (and not water).

119. BD

The pH is the negative $\log_{10}$ of the hydrogen ion concentration. The lower the pH, the higher the hydrogen ion concentration and the higher the acidity. At 37°C the neutral pH (when hydrogen ion concentration equals hydroxyl ion concentration) is 6.8. The plasma pH (7.4) is alkaline. It is, however, more acidic than the pH of the pancreatic juice (8.0). The Henderson–Hasselbalch equation describes the relationship between pH, bicarbonate and the partial pressure of CO_2. By measuring the two latter we can calculate the pH.

120. ACDE

The major buffers in the blood are proteins, mainly haemoglobin and plasma proteins. Haemoglobin has greater buffer value and is present in higher concentration than plasma proteins. The imidazole groups of deoxyhaemoglobin (Hb) dissociates less than those of oxyhaemoglobin (HbO_2), making Hb a weaker acid and therefore a stronger buffer than HbO_2.

121. ACE

Metabolic acidosis occurs when there is excessive acid production (e.g. diabetic ketoacidosis), impaired acid excretion (e.g. renal failure), or excessive alkali loss (e.g. prolonged diarrhoea). In patients with uretero-sigmoid anastomosis there is metabolic acidosis partly due to renal impairment (resulting from previous chronic urinary tract infection), and partly due to the reabsorption of the hydrogen ions secreted in the urine as it passes in the colon. Excessive vomiting causes loss of acidic fluid (gastric secretion) and leads to metabolic alkalosis.

122. ABD

During pregnancy there is hyperventilation, most probably due to progesterone. This acts partly by directly stimulating the respiratory centre and partly by increasing its sensitivity to CO_2. As a result there is a drop in CO_2, but the kidney excretes sufficient bicarbonate to compensate for that and therefore there is no change in pH. The elevated aldosterone levels in pregnancy are necessary for conservation of sodium that would have otherwise been lost due to increased glomerular filtration rate and the natriuretic action of progesterone.

123. ABCE

The ejection fraction is equal to the percentage of the ventricular volume ejected with each stroke and represents a relatively good index of ventricular function. The end-diastolic ventricular volume is about 130 ml. At rest, each ventricle ejects 70–90 ml per stroke, thus giving an ejection fraction of 65%.

124. ABCE

The fetal sleep/activity state affects the heart rate, but is normal and not pathological.

125. BCD

The P–R interval is measured from the beginning of the P wave to the beginning of the QRS complex. It is prolonged in heart block and shortened when the conduction from the atria to the ventricles is abnormally rapid (e.g. Wolff-Parkinson-White syndrome). The P–R interval coincides with the **a** wave in the jugular venous pressure trace. The **v** wave represents the rise in atrial pressure before the tricuspid valve opens during diastole.

126. ACE

Due to mechanical elevation of the diaphragm in pregnancy there is change in the cardiac position and its electrical axis. There is usually a loud third heart sound in pregnancy, but this is an auscultatory finding and not detected on ECG. The P–R interval is not changed.

127. ABDE

The pressure in the right ventricle is dependent on the phase of the cardiac cycle. In systole it should not exceed 35 mmHg and at the end of diastole it is 4 mmHg on average.

128. ABD

The Q–T interval is normally 0.3–0.4 seconds. In the ECG the T wave amplitude varies directly with the serum potassium and the U wave inversely with it. In cases of hypokalaemia there is depression in the S–T segment followed immediately by a prominent U wave. This U wave is often erroneously considered a part of the T, thus falsely prolonging the Q–T interval.

129. CDE

Heart sounds are caused by valve closure; valve opening is normally silent. The second heart sound is due to the closure of the aortic and pulmonary valves. As the left side of the heart contracts before the right side, the aortic component of the second heart sound precedes the pulmonary component, and this splitting is further widened during deep inspiration.

130. ACDE

According to the Frank-Starling law, the energy of contraction is proportional to the initial length of the cardiac muscle. This length is proportional to the amount of blood present in the ventricle at the end of diastole – the ventricular end-diastolic volume (EDV). Factors which affect EDV, and hence ventricular contractility, include atrial systole (contributes one-third of ventricular filling), pumping action of skeletal muscles (increased during exercise), circulating blood volume, venous return, body position, intrathoracic pressure and intrapericardial pressure. Stimulation of the sympathetic nerve supply to the heart increases ventricular contractility without changing the EDV.

131. ABDE

Ritodrine is a beta-adrenergic stimulant which causes increased myocardial contractility. Acidosis, hypercapnia and quinidine cause direct depression of myocardial contractility. Myocardial infarction causes loss of myocardial tissue.

132. CE

During pregnancy cardiac output increases by about 40%. This is mainly due to increased stroke volume; the heart rate increases by only 10%. There is also increased oxygen consumption by body tissues, and hence decreased arteriovenous oxygen gradient. The plasma volume increases by about 43%, and the red cell mass by 17–25%. Consequently there is a reduction in haematocrit and haemoglobin concentration.

133. ABE

Renin, like other hormones, is synthesized as a large preprohormone: preprorenin (406 amino acids). Twenty-three amino acids are removed to form prorenin, and another 43 amino acids are removed to form renin (340 amino acids). It converts angiotensinogen to angiotensin I.

134. BE

Angiotensin II (AII) is an octapeptide. It is formed by the action of angiotensin converting enzyme (ACE) on angiotensin I. ACE is mainly produced in the lungs, but also in the placenta. AII is a very potent vasoconstrictor and causes a rise in systolic and diastolic blood pressure. In normal pregnancy, however, there is reduced sensitivity to AII and, despite its raised levels, there is actually a fall in blood pressure in early pregnancy. AII also stimulates thirst and increases the secretion of aldosterone, vasopressin and antidiuretic hormone. It is metabolized into angiotensin III, which has about 40% of the pressor activity of AII and 100% of its aldosterone-stimulating activity.

135. CD

Central venous pressure and pulmonary capillary wedge pressure do not change during pregnancy. During the second trimester there is about a 40% increase in pulmonary blood flow (PBF) and a 12–19% increase in pulmonary arterial pressure (PAP). The pulmonary vascular resistance (= PAP/PBF) is reduced by up to 25%.

136. BE

The male and female fetuses initially grow at the same rate until the 32nd week of gestation, when the male grows more rapidly. As early as 24–26 weeks the spaces between capillaries and air spaces in the fetal lungs are small enough to allow effective gas exchange in some babies. Also during this time the Type II pneumocytes appear and have the ability to manufacture surfactants. Fetal blood glucose levels are about two-thirds of those of the mother, which facilitates glucose transfer. This is very important as over 90% of fetal energy requirements are obtained from glucose, hence it has been called a 'glucose-dependent parasite'.

137. AC

The fetus has two kinds of adipose tissue: brown and white. Brown fat is especially prominent in hibernating mammals, but makes up a small proportion of total body fat in the fetus, and even a smaller proportion in adults. In white fat, only the blood vessels have sympathetic innervation. In the brown fat the vessels as well as the fat cells themselves have extensive sympathetic innervation. A white adipocyte contains a large single droplet of fat, while the brown adipocyte contains multiple small droplets and is rich in mitochondria. The main function of brown fat is the production of heat through the oxidation of fatty acids within the mitochondria. The heat is released directly (without shivering) by virtue of the 'proton leak' across the mitochondrial membrane.

138. ABCD

During pregnancy there is a resetting of the hypothalamic centres controlling electrolyte levels which leads to a slight fall in the serum levels of sodium and potassium. There is also a fall in calcium and magnesium levels due to the lowered plasma protein concentration. Copper levels, on the other hand, are increased in line with the increased levels of caeruloplasmin. This is due to the action of oestrogen.

139. ABCDE

The Kleihauer acid elution test detects the presence of red cells containing fetal haemoglobin (Hb F). Hb F is more stable than adult haemoglobin (Hb A) and resists acid elution (and alkali denaturation). In the Kleihauer test a film of blood is stained and flooded with a strong acid. Cells containing Hb F retain their haemoglobin and are seen in a sea of 'ghost-like' cells which have lost their Hb A. Conditions in which there is increased Hb F in the circulation will give rise to a positive Kleihauer test. These include hereditary persistent Hb F production, ineffective erythropoiesis (e.g. in haemoglobinopathies) and fetomaternal haemorrhage. The commonest time for fetomaternal haemorrhage is at delivery.

140. ABD

Inspired air has a higher PO_2 and a lower PCO_2 than alveolar air. Expired air is a mixture of alveolar air (350 ml) and inspired air filling the dead space (150 ml), and hence has higher PO_2 and lower PCO_2 than alveolar air. Alveolar ventilation is 350 ml per breath, which is a small proportion of the total volume (2 litres) of alveolar air at the end of expiration (functional residual capacity).

141. BD

Gaseous exchange occurs only in the terminal portions of the airways (alveoli). The gas occupying the rest of the respiratory system is not available for exchange with the pulmonary capillary blood and is termed 'dead space'. The total (physiological) dead space consists of an anatomical component (respiratory system volume exclusive of alveoli) and an alveolar component (alveoli where there is a mismatch between ventilation and perfusion, e.g. heart failure, pulmonary embolism, lung collapse). In healthy individuals the total dead space is almost equal to the anatomical space (150 ml) and there is very little contribution from the alveoli.

142. ABCE

The functional residual capacity is the volume of air left in the lungs at the end of normal resting expiration. It consists of the expiratory reserve volume plus the residual volume. Both these volumes are reduced in normal pregnancy.

143. BD

During pregnancy the respiratory rate and the vital capacity remain unchanged, while the total lung capacity is reduced.

144. ABCDE

The intrapleural pressure is the pressure in the potential space between the visceral pleura and the parietal pleura. At rest it is −3 mmHg and falls down to −6 mmHg at the end of quiet inspiration.

145. BCDE

Lung surfactants are produced by the granular type II pneumocytes and are formed of a mixture of phospholipids (77%), neutral lipids (13%), proteins (8%) and carbohydrates (2%). The protein component greatly enhances the formation of the phospholipid film in the alveoli which reduces the surface tension and prevents their collapse during expiration. Glucocorticoids enhance surfactant production and may be administered to pregnant women who are expected to deliver preterm in order to enhance fetal lung maturity.

146. ABD

During pregnancy ventilation is increased, mainly due to the progesterone effect. Progesterone acts by directly stimulating the respiratory centre as well as increasing its sensitivity (i.e. lowering its threshold) to CO_2. The affinity of maternal haemoglobin to oxygen is progressively decreased in pregnancy to facilitate 'unloading' of oxygen from maternal to fetal blood in the placenta. The airway resistance (as expressed by peak expiratory flow rate and FEV_1) remains unchanged.

147. ACE

The respiratory centre receives input from central chemoreceptors (in the upper medulla) and peripheral chemoreceptors (in the aortic and carotid bodies). The carotid bodies have enormous blood flow per unit tissue (2000 ml per 100 g of tissue per minute, as compared with 420 ml for kidneys and 84 ml for heart muscle) and are, therefore, sensitive to changes in PO_2 rather than oxygen content of the blood. In situations such as anaemia or CO poisoning the amount of oxygen dissolved in the blood is generally normal (despite overall low oxygen content) and the carotid bodies are not stimulated. In cyanide poisoning, on the other hand, oxygen utilization at tissue level is inhibited and the carotid bodies are stimulated.

148. ABCD

Hyperventilation will lead to hypocapnia, which has a direct vasoconstrictor effect on many vessels. It does, however, depress the vasomotor area, so the blood pressure is usually unchanged or only slightly elevated.

149. CDE

The sensitivity of respiratory centres to CO_2 is decreased in trained athletes and with advancing age.

150. ACE

2,3-Diphosphoglycerate (2,3-DPG) is a byproduct of glycolysis and binds to the β chains of deoxyhaemoglobin, causing a shift of the oxygen-haemoglobin dissociation curve to the right, thus reducing affinity. In the presence of Hb F, the concentration of 2,3-DPG is reduced as it binds poorly to the γ chains of the Hb F. Acidosis inhibits red cell glycolysis, causing a fall in the concentration of 2,3-DPG. Red cell 2,3-DPG concentration is increased by thyroxine and growth hormones and in cases of anaemia.

151. BCE

Factors that cause a shift of the oxygen-haemoglobin dissociation curve to the right lead to decreased affinity. These factors include abnormal haemoglobins (e.g. methaemoglobin and Hb S), acidosis (the Bohr effect), hyperthermia and 2,3-DPG.

152. ABD

Plasma contains no carbonic anhydrase and, therefore, carbon dioxide hydration occurs mainly in the red cells. There, bicarbonate ions are formed and diffuse out to plasma in exchange for chloride ions (the chloride shift). Two-thirds of carbon dioxide is transported in plasma as bicarbonate.

153. BCDE

Fetal *haemoglobin* has a low oxygen affinity. However, it binds 2,3-DPG less avidly than does adult haemoglobin. The resulting low levels of 2,3-DPG account for the increased affinity of fetal *blood* for oxygen.

154. AD

Cyanosis (dusky blue discoloration of the tissues) appears when the concentration of reduced haemoglobin (which is dark in colour) is more than 5 g/dl. In CO poisoning the cherry-red colour of carboxymonohaemoglobin is visible in the skin and mucous membranes. In histotoxic hypoxia (e.g. cyanide poisoning) the problem is not in the blood gas content (which is normal) but in the inhibition of tissue oxidative processes. Right to left cardiac shunts cause cyanosis.

155. CDE

The reabsorption of ions and water from the glomerular filtrate occurs mainly in the proximal convoluted tubules. The renal blood flow is normally 1.2 litre/minute. With a haematocrit of 45%, the renal plasma flow is 660 ml/minute.

156. ABD

The fetal kidney is functionally immature and does not have the ability to conserve electrolytes. The fetal urine is, therefore, hypotonic with respect to fetal plasma. Oligohydramnios could be due to reduced fetal urine output (as in intrauterine growth retardation), obstruction of urine flow from the bladder to the amniotic sac (e.g. posterior urethral valve), or increased loss of amniotic fluid (as in cases of rupture of the amniotic membranes).

157. ABC

Plasma osmolality and blood urea concentration are reduced in pregnancy.

158. BCDE

The voiding pressure, as with all other urodynamic pressures, is measured in cm H_2O (and not mmHg).

159. ACDE

Chloride is reabsorbed passively in the proximal convoluted tubules, following sodium and potassium reabsorption. It is also actively reabsorbed in the ascending loop of Henle.

160. ACDE

In the ascending loop of Henle sodium is reabsorbed passively in exchange for chloride ions.

161. CDE

Erythropoietin is a glycoprotein which is formed mainly in the kidney (85%) and also in the liver (15%) during adult life. During fetal and neonatal life, the major site of erythropoiesis as well as erythropoietin production is the liver.

162. BCDE

According to the Laplace law, the pressure in a spherical viscus is equal to twice the wall tension divided by the radius. During bladder filling its wall tension increases, but so does its volume (and radius), and so there is very little rise in intravesical pressure.

163. BD

Gastric acid secretion and plasma protein concentration fall in pregnancy. Hepatic blood flow remains unchanged.

164. ABCE

Glycogen storage in the liver actually increases towards term when the levels reach two to three times those in adult liver. These stores are reduced in growth-retarded fetuses, hence their reduced abdominal circumference on ultrasound scan and relative inability to deal with stress. After delivery, the glycogen content of the liver falls precipitously.

165. ABCE

The presence of fats and carbohydrates in the duodenum inhibits gastric acid and pepsin secretion and gastric motility via gastric inhibitory peptide (GIP) and pepsin secretion.

166. CD

Glucagon and calcitonin inhibit gastrin secretion by the G cells in the gastric antrum. Atropine neither increases nor inhibits gastrin secretion, probably because the transmitter secreted by the postganglionic vagal fibres that innervate the G cells is gastrin releasing peptide (GRP) rather than acetylcholine.

167. BCDE

The pH of the fasting gastric juice is 1.0. The surface mucosa cells secrete mucus (glycoprotein) and bicarbonate which both form an unstirred layer with a pH of 7.0. This layer helps to protect the mucosal surface from damage by gastric acid.

168. AC

The concentration of albumin and gamma-globulin falls during pregnancy, while that of alanine aminotransferase remains unchanged.

169. BCE

After the menopause plasma calcium levels increase. The three principal factors that regulate the plasma calcium concentration are parathyroid hormone (PTH), calcitonin (CT), and 1,25-dihydroxycholecalciferol (vitamin D). PTH increases calcium reabsorption in the kidney and mobilization from the bone by osteoclasts. 1,25-Dihydroxycholecalciferol has the same effects in addition to increasing calcium absorption from the gastrointestinal tract. The net effect of PTH and 1,25-dihydroxycholecalciferol is to increase plasma calcium levels. On the other hand, CT reduces these levels by increasing calcium excretion in the kidney and stimulating bone accretion by osteoblasts.

170. C

Movements of the fetal chest wall as observed by ultrasound are termed 'fetal breathing movements'. They are primarily diaphragmatic and usually decrease in incidence within 72 hours prior to the spontaneous onset of labour, presumably due to increased fetal arterial prostaglandin E levels. They are one of the components of the biophysical profile score, and their presence is taken as an index of fetal health. They are periodic in nature and their absence, on the other hand, particularly over short observation intervals does not necessarily imply fetal hypoxia.

171. BCE

Afferent fibres carrying proprioceptive and enteroceptive sensation from the bladder are mediated via sacral roots S2–4 and ascend in the spinothalamic tracts.

172. CE

During REM sleep the EEG shows rapid, low-voltage irregular activity. Because this pattern replaces the regular alpha rhythm which is thought to be due to synchronized activity of the brain neural elements, it is called 'desynchronization'. During REM sleep there is also a marked reduction in skeletal muscle tone which results from increased activity of the reticular inhibiting area in the medulla. Nocturnal enuresis occurs during non-REM sleep.

173. BD

There are two types of neural response in a reflex arc. At the junctions (between the sense organ and the afferent neuron, at the synapse and at the neuromuscular junction) there is a non-propagated graded response that is proportional to the magnitude of the stimulus. On the other hand, in the parts of the arc specialized for transmission (afferent and efferent axons, muscle membrane) the responses are 'all or none' action potentials.

174. BCDE

The corticospinal tracts are responsible for the initiation of the voluntary movements. The coordination of these movements is a function of the cerebellar system. Eighty per cent of their fibres cross the midline at the pyramidal decussation in the medulla and descend as the lateral corticospinal (pyramidal) tract, and the remaining 20% descend as the ventral corticospinal tract and do not cross the midline until the level at which they synapse with the motor neurons of the anterior horn cells.

175. AE

Pain sensation is transmitted through two types of nerve fibre: myelinated A-delta fibres which are 2–5 μm in diameter, and unmyelinated C fibres which are 0.4–1.2 μm in diameter. Motor nerve fibres (A-beta fibres) are larger (6–14 μm). This is why local anaesthetic agents affect sensory nerves more than they affect motor nerves. The sensory areas in the cerebral cortex are concerned with the discriminative, exact and meaningful interpretation of pain, but perception alone does not require a functioning cortex.

176. BE

The sympathetic outflow starts by preganglionic fibres which leave the spinal cord in the ventral roots of the spinal nerves. These preganglionic fibres pass through a chain of ganglia which lie outside the spinal cord (paravertebral ganglia). This chain extends towards the head to form the cervical ganglion. Not all the preganglionic fibres synapse in these ganglion. Some pass through to synapse at other collateral ganglion (coelic, superior and inferior mesenteric), while others (e.g. sympathetic supply to the uterus) pass through these collateral ganglia to synapse in the organ itself. The adrenal medulla is supplied directly by preganglionic sympathetic fibres, and as such has no postganglionic fibres.

177. ABCE

The cholinergic neurons (i.e. those which have acetylcholine as a chemical transmitter) are: 1) all preganglionic neurons; 2) postganglionic parasympathetic neurons; 3) postganglionic sympathetic neurons to sweat glands; and 4) postganglionic sympathetic vasodilator neurons to the skeletal muscles blood vessels. The remaining postganglionic neurons are noradrenergic.

178. BCE

Noradrenergic stimulation causes contraction of the radial muscle of the iris (mydriasis), while cholinergic stimulation causes contraction of its sphincter muscle (miosis). The muscles of the bladder trigone have a distinct embryological origin from the detrusor, which is why they have different autonomic innervation. The trigone muscles relax in response to cholinergic stimulation and contract with noradrenergic stimulation.

179. ABE

The increased renin secretion is a response to stimulation of beta-1 receptors in the juxtaglomerular cells, while the contraction of the splenic capsule is a response to alpha receptor stimulation.

180. BD

Adrenaline stimulates alpha and beta-1 receptors but not beta-2. Propranolol is a beta blocker and metaraminol is a selective alpha agonist.

181. BCE

Iron is more readily absorbed in the ferrous form, but most dietary iron is in the ferric form. Therefore, substances that enhance the reduction of iron to the ferrous form (such as ascorbic acid) will enhance its absorption. Phosphates (as present in egg yolk) and phytates (as present in cereals) will form insoluble complexes with ferric iron and hence inhibit its absorption.

182. ACD

Ferritin is very stable and not affected by recent ingestion of iron. Only about 25–27% of the total body iron is in the form of ferritin.

183. ABCDE

Although only very little iron is absorbed in the stomach, the gastric secretions dissolve the iron and enhance its absorption in the duodenum. This is why iron deficiency anaemia is a frequent complication of partial gastrectomy.

184. ABDE

The most sensitive indicator of iron deficiency is the mean red cell volume (MCV), and it is the first red cell index to change in iron deficiency anaemia in pregnancy. Total iron binding capacity is raised in iron deficiency anaemia.

185. DE

Prostacyclin is a very potent vasodilator and inhibitor of platelet aggregation. It is synthesized by the endothelium of blood vessels and, during pregnancy, by the placenta, amnion, chorion, decidua and myometrium. Its half-life in blood is only 3 minutes, and therefore its actions are largely local.

186. ABDE

Between 60 and 75% of platelets are in the circulation, and the remainder are mainly in the spleen. Splenectomy, therefore, causes an increase in the platelet count.

187. ACDE

The protein content of lymph varies with the region from which the lymph drains, ranging from 0 g/dl in the choroid plexus to 6.2 g/dl in the liver. The protein content of plasma, however, is higher (about 7 g/dl).

188. ADE

Fibrinolytic activity and antithrombin III concentration are reduced during normal pregnancy.

189. ACE

Tissue plasminogen activators are present in most human tissues with the exception of the placenta. Tranexamic acid is an anti-activator (antiplasminogen) which inhibits the fibrinolytic activity.

190. ABD

The term neonate has reduced levels of proteins S and C; clotting factors II, VII, IX and X; and antithrombin III. It has relatively high haematocrit, blood viscosity and clotting factors V and VIII.

8

Endocrinology

ENDOCRINOLOGY: QUESTIONS

191. Glucagon:

    A. causes glycogenolysis in the muscle.

    B. is secreted by the delta cells of the islets of Langerhans in the pancreas.

    C. is released in response to exercise.

    D. stimulates gluconeogenesis.

    E. stimulates the secretion of growth hormone.

192. Insulin facilitates glucose uptake in:

    A. brain tissue.

    B. adipose tissue.

    C. red blood cells.

    D. leukocytes.

    E. the pituitary gland.

193. Insulin release is stimulated by:

    A. glucose.

    B. somatostatin.

    C. diazoxide.

    D. glucagon.

    E. amino acids.

194. Somatostatin:

    A. is produced by delta cells of the pancreatic islets.

    B. secretion is stimulated by amino acids.

    C. stimulates gut motility.

    D. inhibits glucagon release.

    E. inhibits growth hormone release.

195. Hormones produced by the hypothalamus include:

    A. luteinizing hormone.

    B. oxytocin.

    C. somatostatin.

    D. gonadotrophin releasing hormone.

    E. thyroid stimulating hormone.

196. Alpha melanocyte stimulating hormone:

    A. is produced by the anterior lobe of the pituitary gland.

    B. is the main type of melanocyte stimulating hormone in human adults.

    C. contains 13 amino acid residues.

    D. has similar chemical structure to the adrenocorticotrophic hormone (ACTH).

    E. increases melatonin synthesis.

197. The pineal gland:

    A. is relatively larger in the infant than it is in the adult.

    B. secretes melatonin into the cerebrospinal fluid.

    C. arises from the floor of the third ventricle.

    D. is innervated by noradrenaline-secreting postganglionic sympathetic nerves.

    E. contains neuroglial cells.

198. Hormones produced by the anterior lobe of the pituitary gland include:

    A. prolactin.

    B. thyroid stimulating hormone.

    C. oestradiol.

    D. growth hormone.

    E. oxytocin.

199. Follicle stimulating hormone (FSH):

 A. is a glycoprotein.

 B. is produced by the chromophil cells of the anterior lobe of the pituitary gland.

 C. stimulates the interstitial cells of Leydig in the male.

 D. has alpha-subunits which are the product of the same gene that controls the alpha-subunits of luteinizing hormone (LH) and thyroid stimulating hormone (TSH).

 E. serum levels are increased during the climacteric.

200. Inhibin:

 A. inhibits FSH secretion.

 B. is produced by the interstitial cells of Leydig in the male.

 C. is produced by the granulosa cells in the female.

 D. is a polypeptide.

 E. has a direct action on the pituitary gland.

201. Luteinizing hormone (LH):

 A. is bound to plasma proteins.

 B. secretion is stimulated by rising levels of oestrogen.

 C. production is increased by sustained continuous adminis-tration of gonadotrophin releasing hormone analogues.

 D. stimulates testosterone production in the female.

 E. surge occurs within 36 hours after ovulation.

202. Ovulation:

 A. occurs from alternate ovaries in successive cycles.

 B. is preceded by a marked rise in serum oestrogen.

 C. does not occur during the first 6 postnatal weeks.

 D. is followed by a marked rise in serum progesterone.

 E. is always followed by menstruation.

203. During the second trimester of normal pregnancy there is a progressive increase in the production of:

 A. human chorionic gonadotrophin.

 B. oestriol.

    C. human placental lactogen.

    D. luteinizing hormone.

    E. progesterone.

204. Human growth hormone:

    A. is protein bound in the plasma.

    B. stimulates carbohydrates oxidation.

    C. has lactogenic activity.

    D. is produced by the acidophil cells of the anterior lobe of the pituitary gland.

    E. secretion is markedly increased during pregnancy.

205. Growth hormone secretion is increased by:

    A. medroxyprogesterone.

    B. oestrogen.

    C. REM sleep.

    D. hypoglycaemia.

    E. androgen.

206. Growth hormone secretion is decreased by:

    A. the ingestion of a protein meal.

    B. exercise.

    C. glucagon.

    D. apomorphine.

    E. vasopressin.

207. Prolactin:

    A. is necessary for the initiation of lactation.

    B. is produced by the basophil cells of the anterior lobe of the pituitary gland.

    C. secreting cells increase markedly in number during pregnancy.

    D. secretion is under the control of hypothalamic gonado-trophin releasing hormone.

    E. stimulates the production of lactalbumin in the breast postnatally.

208. Prolactin secretion is increased by:

    A. sleep.

    B. bromocriptine.

    C. somatostatin.

    D. physical exercise.

    E. sexual intercourse.

209. Relaxin hormone is found in:

    A. semen.

    B. the endometrium during the proliferative phase of the menstrual cycle.

    C. chorionic cytotrophoblasts.

    D. the placental plate.

    E. the corpus luteum.

210. Oxytocin:

    A. is a nonapeptide.

    B. is synthesized in the posterior lobe of the pituitary gland.

    C. receptors in the uterus increase towards the end of pregnancy.

    D. secretion is stimulated by alcohol.

    E. has some antidiuretic action.

211. Vasopressin secretion is increased by:

    A. alcohol.

    B. physical exercise.

    C. increased extracellular fluid volume.

    D. angiotensin II.

    E. morphine.

212. Vasopressin:

    A. increases the permeability of the renal collecting tubular cells to water.

    B. secretion is increased in response to haemorrhage.

    C. is an octapeptide.

    D. may elevate arterial blood pressure by direct action on the arteriolar smooth muscles.

    E. secretion is increased by nausea.

213. Lactation:

    A. is initiated postnatally in response to the rising levels of oestrogen.

    B. does not occur in the absence of maternal pituitary growth hormone.

    C. can inhibit ovulation.

    D. is inhibited by progesterone.

    E. is inhibited by bromocriptine.

214. The follicular phase of the ovarian cycle is associated with:

    A. a proliferative pattern in the endometrium.

    B. the commencement of the first meiotic division in the oocyte.

    C. proliferation of the mammary ducts.

    D. increased basal body temperature.

    E. a peak in oestradiol plasma levels.

215. During the menstrual cycle:

    A. menstrual blood loss is predominantly arterial.

    B. menstrual blood loss more than 80 ml is abnormal.

    C. ovulation is an essential prerequisite for menstruation.

    D. variations in the cycle length are mainly due to variations in the length of the secretory phase.

    E. menstrual blood loss does not normally contain clots.

216. Sex hormone binding globulin binds:

    A. androstenedione.

    B. testosterone.

    C. progesterone.

    D. oestradiol.

    E. cortisol.

217. Sex hormone binding globulin:

    A. binds testosterone with a greater affinity than does albumin.

    B. binds about 95% of circulating testosterone in the female.

    C. concentration is reduced during pregnancy.

    D. concentration is increased in hyperthyroidism.

    E. concentration is reduced with oestrogen therapy.

218. Progesterone:

    A. is derived from cholesterol.

    B. secretion from the corpus luteum reaches a maximum on day 21 following luteinizing hormone (LH) surge in a 28-day menstrual cycle.

    C. is excreted in the urine as pregnanediol glucuronide.

    D. decreases the number of oestrogen receptors in the endometrium.

    E. enters the target cells by simple diffusion.

219. Oestrogen:

    A. increases the secretion of angiotensinogen.

    B. reduces the number of progesterone receptors in the endometrium.

    C. is responsible for pubic hair growth in the female at puberty.

    D. is responsible for pigmentation of the areola of the breast at puberty.

    E. is produced by the corpus luteum.

220. Testosterone:

    A. causes an increase in scalp hair.

    B. secretion is under the control of luteinizing hormone.

    C. is excreted in the urine as 17-oxosteroids.

    D. is produced by the ovarian stroma.

    E. binds to the same intracellular receptors as does dihydrotestosterone.

221. Atrial natriuretic peptide:

    A. causes an increase in arterial blood pressure.

    B. inhibits vasopressin secretion.

    C. inhibits renin secretion.

    D. plasma concentration is decreased on rising from the supine to the standing position.

    E. increases the glomerular filtration rate.

222. Sertoli cells secrete:

    A. testosterone.

    B. androstenedione.

    C. inhibin.

    D. androgen-binding protein.

    E. Müllerian inhibiting substance.

223. Growth and maturation of the breast at puberty is promoted by:

    A. oestrogen.

    B. progesterone.

    C. insulin.

    D. cortisol.

    E. parathyroid hormone.

224. Testosterone:

    A. when administered systemically stimulates spermatogenesis.

    B. inhibits luteinizing hormone secretion.

    C. is secreted from the male fetus gonads during the first trimester.

    D. causes sodium and water retention.

    E. is secreted by the adrenal medulla.

225. The menarche is usually:

    A. delayed in undernourished girls.

    B. the first sign of puberty.

    C. followed by ovulatory cycles.

D. related to bone age more closely than it is related to chrono-
logical age.

E. between the ages of 11 and 15 years in about 90% of girls in
Western Europe.

226. **Follicle stimulating hormone (FSH) serum levels are
markedly raised in:**

A. postmenopausal women.

B. women taking the combined oral contraceptive pill.

C. prepubertal girls following gonadectomy.

D. pregnancy.

E. Sheehan's syndrome.

227. **Conditions associated with hypogonadotrophic
hypogonadism include:**

A. Turner's syndrome.

B. premature ovarian failure.

C. Kallmann's syndrome.

D. anorexia nervosa.

E. Klinefelter's syndrome.

228. **Polycystic ovarian disease is associated with raised levels of:**

A. follicle stimulated hormone.

B. luteinizing hormone.

C. progesterone.

D. testosterone.

E. sex hormone binding globulin.

229. **Epidermal growth factor:**

A. is a steroid hormone.

B. augments FSH action on granulosa cells.

C. augments granulosa cells proliferation.

D. stimulates insulin-like growth factor-I (IGF-I) production.

E. is produced in the ovary.

230. Insulin-like growth factor-I (IGF-I):

  A. is synthesized in the liver.

  B. synthesis in the granulosa cells is enhanced by growth hormone.

  C. inhibits androgen production from the theca cells.

  D. is a peptide.

  E. is protein-bound in the plasma.

231. The postmenopausal state is associated with a rise in:

  A. serum phosphate.

  B. urinary calcium creatinine ratio.

  C. serum alkaline phosphatase.

  D. urinary hydroxyproline.

  E. serum calcium.

232. Recognized consequences of insulin excess include:

  A. weakness.

  B. tremors.

  C. palpitations.

  D. dizziness.

  E. confusion.

233. Hypoglycaemia causes increased secretion of:

  A. epinephrine.

  B. prolactin.

  C. growth hormone.

  D. glucagon.

  E. cortisol.

234. Insulin deficiency leads to:

  A. diuresis.

  B. reduced plasma amino acids.

  C. ketonuria.

  D. increased plasma free fatty acids.

  E. increased plasma cholesterol.

235. In Turner's syndrome there is:

    A. low level of growth hormone.

    B. congenital absence of oocytes.

    C. normal intellectual ability.

    D. normal level of insulin-like growth factor-I (IGF-I).

    E. higher incidence of osteoporosis.

236. Hyperprolactinaemia is a recognized side-effect of:

    A. reserpine.

    B. sulpiride.

    C. haloperidol.

    D. methyldopa.

    E. metoclopramide.

237. In a normal ovulatory menstrual cycle:

    A. FSH levels start to rise during the luteal phase of the previous cycle.

    B. only one follicle is usually recruited.

    C. ovulation occurs 36 hours following LH peak.

    D. both FSH and LH levels rise prior to ovulation.

    E. LH is important for follicular development during the follicular phase.

238. Corticosterone:

    A. is secreted by all three cortical zones of the adrenal gland.

    B. has 21 carbon atoms.

    C. has glucocorticoid activity of similar potency to that of cortisol.

    D. is secreted in a similar concentration to that of cortisol.

    E. increases hepatic gluconeogenesis.

239. There are 21 carbon atoms in the structure of:

    A. aldosterone.

    B. progesterone.

    C. oestradiol.

    D. testosterone.

    E. cortisol.

240. The fetal zone of the adrenal cortex:

    A. is under pituitary control.

    B. persists till puberty.

    C. secretes dehydroepiandrosterone sulphate (DHAS).

    D. is derived from mesoderm.

    E. forms almost 80% of the fetal adrenal cortex during intrauterine life.

241. Adrenocorticotrophic hormone (ACTH):

    A. secretion is increased in congenital adrenal hyperplasia.

    B. is secreted from the basophil cells of the anterior pituitary gland.

    C. stimulates the conversion of cholesterol to pregnenolone.

    D. secretion is under hypothalamic control.

    E. is the main hormone controlling aldosterone secretion.

242. Glucocorticoids lead to an increase in the number of circulating:

    A. red blood cells.

    B. platelets.

    C. lymphocytes.

    D. neutrophils.

    E. eosinophils.

243. Cortisol:

    A. exerts an anti-insulin action on the heart.

    B. inhibits protein synthesis in the liver.

    C. increases urinary calcium excretion.

    D. increases sodium reabsorption by the renal tubules.

    E. inhibits glucose uptake by striated muscles.

244. During normal pregnancy there is an increase in the plasma levels of:

    A. aldosterone.

    B. total cortisol.

    C. free cortisol.

    D. catecholamines.

    E. growth hormone.

245. During normal pregnancy there is an increase in:

    A. glucagon plasma levels.

    B. insulin resistance.

    C. postprandial insulin levels.

    D. the incidence of glycosuria.

    E. the rate with which insulin crosses the placenta.

246. During normal pregnancy there is an increase in the plasma levels of:

    A. oestriol.

    B. thyroid stimulating hormone (TSH).

    C. melanocyte stimulating hormone (MSH).

    D. human placental lactogen.

    E. albumin.

247. Aldosterone:

    A. increases the reabsorption of sodium from sweat.

    B. leads to a decrease in urine acidity.

    C. secretion is stimulated by angiotensin II.

    D. secretion is more sensitive to changes in plasma sodium concentration than it is to changes in plasma potassium concentration.

    E. secretion is inhibited by atrial natriuretic peptide.

248. The following increase the secretion of both aldosterone and cortisol from the adrenal cortex:

    A. surgery.

    B. haemorrhage.

    C. standing position.

    D. anxiety.

    E. high potassium intake.

249. **Adrenocorticotrophic hormone (ACTH):**

    A. secretion has a diurnal (circadian) rhythm.

    B. is a polypeptide.

    C. mediates the stress-related increase in glucocorticoid secretion.

    D. decreases the sensitivity of the adrenal gland to further doses of ACTH.

    E. stimulates androgen secretion from the adrenal gland.

250. **Corticosteroid-binding globulin (CBG):**

    A. binds over 90% of circulating cortisol.

    B. levels are decreased in pregnancy.

    C. is synthesized in the liver.

    D. levels are increased in nephrosis.

    E. binds corticosterone to a lesser degree than it binds cortisol.

251. **Androgens from the adrenal cortex:**

    A. are under the control of pituitary gonadotrophins.

    B. form almost 90% of the circulating androgens in the normal female.

    C. are excreted as 17-oxogenic steroids.

    D. play an important role in the initiation of puberty in the female.

    E. are synthesized in the zona reticularis.

252. **Hypofunction of the adrenal cortex may lead to:**

    A. a decrease in cardiac size.

    B. skin pigmentation.

    C. hyperglycaemia.

    D. amenorrhoea.

    E. polyuria.

253. Congenital adrenal hyperplasia is associated with:

A. autosomal recessive pattern of inheritance.

B. 21 beta-hydroxylase deficiency as the commonest defect.

C. precocious puberty.

D. male pseudohermaphroditism.

E. a salt-losing syndrome.

254. The adrenal medulla:

A. is essential for life.

B. secretes dopamine.

C. is derived from mesoderm.

D. is supplied by the greater splanchnic nerve.

E. constitutes about one-third of the mass of the adrenal gland.

255. Glucocorticoids inhibit:

A. the combination of antigen and antibody.

B. the effects of histamine in allergic reactions.

C. phospholipase A_2.

D. fibroblastic activity.

E. antibody levels.

256. Adrenaline:

A. is synthesized from tyrosine.

B. is the precursor of noradrenaline.

C. stimulates glycogenolysis.

D. inhibits insulin release from the pancreas

E. is metabolized into vanillylmandelic acid.

257. The secretion of adrenaline from the adrenal medulla is increased in response to:

A. hypoglycaemia.

B. sleep.

C. ketoacidosis.

D. cigarette smoking.

E. physical exercise.

258. By the end of the first trimester the fetus is able to synthesize:

    A. oxytocin.

    B. luteinizing hormone.

    C. growth hormone.

    D. prolactin.

    E. testosterone.

259. Thyroxine (T_4) is:

    A. less potent than reverse tri-iodothyronine (rT_3).

    B. more protein bound than tri-iodothyronine (T_3)

    C. bound to thyroxine binding prealbumin in the plasma.

    D. secreted in greater proportions than tri-iodothyronine.

    E. converted to tri-iodothyronine in peripheral tissue.

260. Iodide trapping by the thyroid gland:

    A. occurs against a concentration gradient.

    B. is stimulated by thyroid stimulating hormone (TSH).

    C. is inhibited by propylthiouracil.

    D. cannot occur until it is oxidized into iodine.

    E. is inhibited by perchlorate.

261. Thyroid stimulation hormone (TSH):

    A. is a glycoprotein.

    B. secretion is inhibited by somatostatin.

    C. levels are increased in normal pregnancy.

    D. has beta subunits similar to those of luteinizing hormone.

    E. secretion is stimulated by stress.

262. Active transport of iodide occurs in:

    A. the placenta.

    B. the fetal thyroid gland.

    C. the mammary gland.

    D. the salivary gland.

    E. the gastric mucosa.

263. Thyroid hormones:

   A. stimulate the oxygen consumption of metabolically active tissue.
   B. cross the placenta.
   C. stimulate the metabolism of the non-pregnant uterus.
   D. increase carbohydrate absorption from the gastrointestinal tract.
   E. increase the circulating cholesterol levels.

264. Thyroxine binding globulin levels are increased:

   A. during intrauterine life.
   B. by glucocorticoids.
   C. during pregnancy.
   D. by danazol.
   E. by androgens.

265. Regarding thyroid function in the fetus and neonate:

   A. thyroxine is secreted by the end of the first trimester.
   B. the control of fetal thyroid is dependent upon maternal TSH.
   C. reverse T_3 is secreted in relatively large amounts.
   D. neonatal TSH levels are decreased in the first day of life.
   E. long-acting thyroid stimulants (LATS) cross the placenta.

266. During pregnancy there is normally an increase in:

   A. plasma iodide levels.
   B. the size of the thyroid gland.
   C. protein-bound iodine levels.
   D. free thyroxine levels.
   E. total tri-iodothyronine levels.

267. During pregnancy there is an increase in the plasma levels of:

   A. deoxycorticosterone.
   B. dehydroepiandrosterone sulphate.
   C. testosterone.

  D. androstenedione.

  E. alkaline phosphatase.

268. **The placenta secretes:**

  A. alpha-fetoprotein.

  B. oestradiol.

  C. oestriol.

  D. human chorionic gonadotrophin.

  E. 16-hydroxy dehydroepiandrosterone sulphate.

269. **In normal pregnancy:**

  A. oestrogen production is shared in equal proportions between the placenta and the maternal ovary.

  B. the predominant oestrogen is oestriol.

  C. most of the weight gain is during the first trimester.

  D. there is relative refractoriness to the pressor effects of angiotensin II.

  E. there is hypertrophy of the musculature of the Fallopian tubes.

270. **The decidua:**

  A. secretes prolactin.

  B. secretes relaxin.

  C. parietalis and decidua capsularis fuse at about 6 weeks intrauterine life.

  D. is the endometrium of pregnancy.

  E. basalis forms the basal plate of the placenta.

▌ ENDOCRINOLOGY: ANSWERS

191. CDE

Glucagon is secreted by the alpha cells of the islets of Langerhans in the pancreas. It is glycogenolytic (in the liver but not in the muscle), gluconeogenic, lipolytic and ketogenic. It also stimulates the secretion of growth hormone, insulin and pancreatic somatostatin.

192. BDE

Insulin facilitates glucose uptake in most body tissues except for the hepatic cells, brain tissue, kidney tubules, intestinal mucosa and red blood cells. This occurs by increasing the number of glucose transporters in the cell membrane. These transporters are a family of related proteins that carry glucose across cell membranes.

193. ADE

Somatostatin and diazoxide inhibit the release of insulin.

194. ABDE

Somatostatin inhibits gastric emptying, gastric acid secretion, gut motility and gall bladder contraction.

195. BCD

The hypothalamus produces gonadotrophin releasing hormone, corticotrophin releasing hormone, growth hormone releasing hormone, growth hormone release-inhibiting hormone (somatostatin), thyrotrophic hormone releasing hormone, prolactin inhibiting factor (dopamine), oxytocin and vasopressin.

196. CD

Alpha melanocyte stimulating hormone (MSH) is produced by the intermediate lobe of the pituitary gland. This lobe is rudimentary in humans, and alpha MSH does not appear to be secreted in adults. Alpha MSH is made up of the first 13 amino acid residues of ACTH and, hence, ACTH has considerable MSH activity. MSH increases melanin (and not melatonin) synthesis.

197. ABDE

The pineal gland arises from the roof of the third ventricle as an upgrowth under the posterior end of the corpus callosum. In infants the pineal gland is large but begins to involute before puberty when small concretions of calcium phosphate and carbonate appear in its tissue. These concretions are responsible for the gland's radio-opacity, often visible on skull X-ray films in adults.

198. ABD

Other anterior pituitary hormones include: follicle stimulating hormone, luteinizing hormone and adrenocorticotrophic hormone.

199. ABDE

In the male FSH helps maintain the spermatogenic epithelium by stimulating Sertoli cells, while LH (also called interstitial cell stimulating hormone–ICSH) stimulates the interstitial cells which produce androgens.

200. ACDE

Inhibin is produced by the Sertoli cells in the male.

201. BD

Gonadotrophin releasing hormone (GnRH) is normally produced in a pulsatile fashion. Continuous administration of exogenous GnRH analogues leads initially to increased production of LH and FSH (flare-up effect), followed by decreased production when this continuous administration is sustained (down regulation). LH surge occurs within 36 hours prior to ovulation.

202. BD

Ovulation occurs from both ovaries in a random fashion. It has been documented as early as 25 days postnatally and contraception is needed from the end of the third postnatal week. Ovulation is often – but not always – followed by menstruation. If followed by pregnancy or associated with menstrual flow obstruction (e.g. imperforate hymen), menstruation will not follow ovulation.

203. BCE

From the beginning of pregnancy the production of luteinizing hormone is reduced due to the negative feedback from the rising levels of oestrogen. Human chorionic gonadotrophin production peaks during the end of the first trimester and then drops to reach a plateau at the middle of the second trimester.

204. ACD

Human growth hormone has marked structural similarity with prolactin and human placental lactogen (HPL). Hence, prolactin and HPL have growth-promoting activity and growth hormone has lactogenic activity. During pregnancy the secretion of growth hormone from the maternal pituitary gland is not increased and may actually be decreased because of the increased levels of HPL. Growth hormone has anti-insulin activity and decreases both insulin receptors and carbohydrate oxidation in the tissues.

205. BDE

Human growth hormone secretion is decreased by medroxy-progesterone, REM sleep, glucose, free fatty acids and cortisol.

206. ALL FALSE

All these factors increase the secretion of growth hormone.

207. ACE

Prolactin is produced by the acidophil cells of the anterior lobe of the pituitary gland and its secretion is under the control of a hypothalamic inhibiting factor (dopamine). In addition, thyrotrophin (TRH) increases prolactin secretion and the presence of a hypothalamic prolactin releasing hormone (TRH or a similar hormone) has been suggested but not yet proven.

208. ADE

Bromocriptine (a dopamine agonist) decreases prolactin secretion and is used in the treatment of hyperprolactinaemia. Somatostatin has no effect on the secretion of prolactin.

209. ACDE

Relaxin is found in the endometrium of the secretory – but not the proliferative – phase of the menstrual cycle.

210. ACE

Oxytocin is synthesized in the nerve cells of the hypothalamic (supraoptic and paraventricular) nuclei and carried down the nerve axons in the pituitary stalk to the posterior lobe of the pituitary gland where it is secreted. Alcohol inhibits the secretion of oxytocin and, in the past, has been used as a tocolytic to reduce uterine contractions in preterm labour.

211. BDE

Alcohol and increased extracellular fluid volume inhibit vasopressin secretion.

212. ABDE

Vasopressin, like oxytocin, is a nonapeptide. Its effect on blood pressure is evident in large doses and the amount of endogenous hormone in the circulation does not normally affect blood pressure.

213. CE

During pregnancy oestrogen and prolactin synergize in producing breast growth, but oestrogen antagonizes the milk-producing effect of prolactin on the breast. After delivery of the placenta, there is an abrupt decline in the circulating levels of oestrogen which leads to the initiation of lactation. In fact, oestrogen was used in the past to suppress lactation (now obsolete because of the risk of thromboembolism). Normal breast growth and lactation can occur in dwarfs with congenital growth hormone deficiency. Progesterone does not inhibit lactation and is widely used for contraception in lactating women (e.g. progesterone-only oral pill and the long acting injectable medroxyprogesterone).

214. ACE

The first meiotic division of the oocyte commences *in utero*. This division is arrested during prophase and is only completed at ovulation to produce a secondary oocyte and a polar body. The secondary oocyte will undergo the second meiotic division only after fertilization. The increase in basal body temperature occurs in the luteal phase of ovulatory cycles due to the thermogenic effect of progesterone.

215. ABE

Menstruation occurs in ovulatory and anovulatory cycles. The length of the secretory phase is remarkably constant at about 14 days, and the variations seen in the cycle length are mainly due to variations in the length of the proliferative phase.

216. ABD

Two per cent of circulating progesterone is free, 18% is bound to corticosteroid binding globulin, and 80% is bound to albumin. The corresponding values for cortisol are 4%, 90% and 6%.

217. AD

Sex hormone binding globulin (SHBG) binds testosterone with an affinity about 50 000 times greater than albumin does. In the female 1% of circulating testosterone is free, 60% is bound to SHBG and 19% is bound to albumin. SHBG concentration is increased during pregnancy and with oestrogen therapy.

218. ACDE

The maximum secretion of progesterone from the corpus luteum occurs about day 8 after LH surge (day 21 of a 28-day cycle).

219. ADE

Oestrogen increases the number of progesterone receptors in the endometrium; hence progesterone will only act on an oestrogen-primed endometrium. Pubic and axillary hair growth at puberty is due primarily to androgens produced by the adrenal cortex.

220. BCDE

Although body hair is increased by testosterone, scalp hair is decreased.

221. BCDE

Atrial natriuretic peptide (ANP) lowers arterial blood pressure. The decrease in ANP plasma concentration on rising is due to the decrease in central venous pressure.

222. CDE

Testosterone and androstenedione are secreted by the interstitial cells of Leydig.

223. ABCDE

Growth hormone also promotes breast maturation at puberty. In rats, some prolactin is also needed for breast development at puberty, but it is not known whether prolactin is necessary in humans.

224. BCD

Naturally secreted testosterone (from the Leydig cells) bathes the seminiferous tubules and provides the high local concentration to the Sertoli cells that is necessary to stimulate spermatogenesis. On the other hand, systematically administered testosterone does not raise the levels in the testes to as great a degree, and it also inhibits LH secretion. Consequently, the net effect of systematically administered testosterone is to inhibit spermatogenesis. The adrenal cortex (and not the medulla) secretes testosterone.

225. ADE

In over 50% of girls, the first sign of puberty is thelarche (the development of breasts), followed by pubarche (the development of pubic and axillary hair) and then by menarche (the first menstrual period). The menstrual cycles following menarche are often irregular and anovulatory.

226. A

Pregnant women and those taking the combined oral contraceptive pill have reduced levels of FSH due to the negative feedback from the raised oestrogen levels. In contrast to the situation in adulthood, gonadectomy from birth to puberty causes little or no increase in gonadotrophin secretion. Sheehan's syndrome is postpartum panhypopituitarism (usually secondary to severe hypotension resulting from postpartum haemorrhage) and leads to hypogonadotrophic hypogonadism.

227. CD

Turner's syndrome (45,X), premature ovarian failure and Klinefelter's syndrome (47,XXY) are examples of hypergonadotrophic hypogonadism.

228. BD

Patients with polycystic ovarian disease (PCOD) have raised levels of LH, with normal or low levels of FSH, leading to the characteristic raised LH/FSH ratio. Androgens (testosterone, androstenedione) are also raised, which suppress the production of SHBG. These patients are often anovulatory, hence the low progesterone levels.

229. CD

Epidermal growth factor is a peptide containing 53 amino acids and was first isolated from the rat salivary glands. It inhibits FSH action on granulosa cells.

230. ABDE

IGF-I acts on the theca cells to augment androgen production either directly or by enhancing LH activity.

231. ABCDE

All these changes are due to increased resorption of calcium and phosphorus from bone leading to a negative calcium and phosphorus balance. Oestrogen administration can reverse these changes, presumably due to inhibition of bone resorption.

232. ABCDE

All the known consequences of insulin excess are manifestations, directly or indirectly, of the effects of hypoglycaemia on the nervous system. Hypoglycaemia is a potent stimulus to catecholamine secretion, which causes tremors and palpitations.

233. ACDE

The main two hormones that antagonize the fall in blood glucose level are epinephrine and glucagon. Cortisol, norepinephrine and growth hormone are also secreted in response to hyperglycaemia, but their action is supplementary.

234. ACDE

Insulin deficiency (as in diabetes mellitus) leads to increased protein catabolism and, consequently, to increased plasma amino acids and nitrogen loss in the urine.

235. CDE

In Turner's syndrome there is normal level of growth hormone. IGF-I level is normal or slightly elevated. The oocytes are formed *in utero* but fail to surround themselves with granulosa cells and, therefore, undergo atresia at a very rapid rate.

236. ABCDE

A and D are dopamine depleting agents while the other drugs are dopamine receptor blocking agents.

237. ADE

Each cycle many follicles are recruited but only one is selected for dominance and ovulation. Ovulation occurs 34–36 hours following the onset of LH surge and 10–12 hours after the LH peak. LH plays an important role in early follicular development and women who suffer from hypogonadotrophic hypogonadism need both FSH and LH for induction of ovulation.

238. ABE

Corticosterone has almost one-third of the glucocorticoid activity of cortisol. The ratio of secreted cortisol to corticosterone is approximately 7.

239. ABE

Oestrogens have 18 carbon atoms in their structure and androgens have 19. Progesterone, mineralocorticoids and glucocorticoids have 21 carbon atoms.

240. ACDE

The fetal zone of the adrenal cortex undergoes rapid regression after birth. The DHAS it secretes acts as a substrate for oestriol synthesis by the feto-placental unit in pregnancy.

241. ABCD

The main control of aldosterone secretion is via the renin-angiotensin system.

242. ABD

Glucocorticoids inhibit lymphocyte proliferation and thus reduce their number. They also reduce the number of circulating eosinophils by increasing their sequestration in the spleen and lungs. The number of circulating basophils is also reduced. The total white cell count, however, is increased due to an increase in the neutrophils.

243. CDE

Cortisol exerts an anti-insulin action in peripheral tissues. The brain and heart, however, are spared. Although the actions of cortisol are generally catabolic, on the liver they are anabolic: increasing hepatic gluconeogenesis, protein synthesis and glycogen formation.

244. ABC

The levels of catecholamines and growth hormone do not change significantly during pregnancy.

245. BCD

Pregnancy has no effect on the alpha cells of the pancreatic islets and glucagon levels are virtually unchanged during pregnancy. Insulin does not cross the placenta.

246. ACD

During pregnancy TSH remains unchanged and albumin levels are reduced.

247. ACE

Aldosterone increases the reabsorption of sodium from the urine, sweat, saliva and gastric juice. The reabsorbed sodium is exchanged for potassium and hydrogen ions, thus increasing the urine acidity. Aldosterone secretion is more sensitive to changes in plasma potassium level than sodium level. An increase of just 1 mEq/L in potassium will increase aldosterone production, while a decrease of at least 20 mEq/L in sodium is needed to produce the same effect.

248. ABD

High potassium intake and standing position increase the secretion of aldosterone, but not cortisol.

249. ABCE

ACTH increases not only the glucocorticoid secretion from the adrenal cortex but also the sensitivity of the adrenal to subsequent doses of ACTH.

250. ACE

CBG levels are increased in pregnancy (due to the effect of oestrogen on the liver) and decreased in nephrosis. It is the free (unbound) fraction of cortisol that is biologically active. This explains why pregnant women have high total plasma cortisol levels without symptoms of glucocorticoid excess.

251. DE

The secretion of adrenal androgens is under the control of ACTH and possibly another, yet undefined, pituitary factor (adrenal androgen-stimulating hormone). It is not controlled by the pituitary gonadotrophins (FSH, LH). Adrenal androgen contributes about 50% of circulating androgen in normal females and is excreted as 17-oxosteroids. 17-Oxogenic steroids are the metabolites of glucocorticoids.

252. ABDE

In hypofunction of the adrenal cortex (Addison's disease) there is chronic hypotension leading to a reduction in cardiac size. ACTH levels are elevated and, through its MSH-like activity, there is hyperpigmentation. The polyuria is due to sodium diuresis. There is also hypoglycaemia.

253. ABCE

Due to the excessive secretion of androgens in severe CAH there may be precocious puberty in males and 'female' pseudohermaphroditism in females.

It is important to understand properly the nomenclature of hermaphroditism: 'male' or 'female' refer to the genetic sex; 'pseudo' or 'true' refer to the presence of one type of gonads (testis or ovary) or both, respectively; and hermaphroditism refers to the imperfect sexual differentiation into either male or female.

254. BDE

The adrenal medulla is not essential for life, unlike the adrenal cortex. Embryologically, the medulla is derived from the neuroectoderm.

255. CDE

In allergic reactions antibodies combine with antigens, provoking the release of histamine from mast cells, which in turn causes many of the symptoms of allergy. Glucocorticoids do not affect the combination of antigen with antibody and have no influence on the effects of histamine once it is released, but they prevent histamine release.

256. ACDE

Noradrenaline is the precursor of adrenaline and both are synthesized from the amino acid tyrosine.

257. ACDE

The secretion of adrenaline and, to a lesser extent, noradrenaline is reduced during sleep.

258. ABCDE

All these hormones have been isolated from the human fetus by about 10 weeks gestation.

259. BCDE

The thyroid gland secretes more T_4 than T_3. However, T_3 is more active than T_4, whereas rT_3 is inactive. Moreover, T_3 is less protein bound than T_4. This is why T_3 is responsible for more peripheral activities than T_4.

260. ABE

Iodide trapping by the thyroid cells is an active transport mechanism occurring against a thyroid/plasma iodide ratio of over 100. Iodide is transported as such and then oxidized into iodine before reacting with tyrosine to form monoiodotyrosine. Perchlorate and other related anions inhibit iodide trapping. Propylthiouracil exerts its antithyroid action by preventing the oxidation of iodide, the release of T_3 and T_4, and the peripheral conversion of T_4 into T_3.

261. AB

TSH levels are virtually unchanged during normal pregnancy. It has two subunits: alpha and beta. The alpha subunits are identical in structure to those of FSH and LH and differ only slightly from those of hCG. The beta subunits, on the other hand, are different in all those hormones. TSH secretion is inhibited by stress through its inhibitory effect on TRH.

262. ABCDE

Radioactive iodine should not be administered during pregnancy as it is transported across the placenta and concentrated in the fetal thyroid gland – even more avidly than in the maternal thyroid. This may induce hypothyroidism in the fetus or cause thyroid cancer later in the child's life. Also, it should not be given to breast-feeding mothers as it is secreted in high concentration in breast milk.

263. ABD

Thyroid hormones cross the placenta, but only in small amounts. They stimulate the metabolism of many tissues, with the exception of the adult brain, uterus, testis, lymph nodes, spleen and anterior pituitary. They are, however, essential for normal menstruation and fertility. They lower the circulating cholesterol levels due to increased formation of LDL receptors.

264. AC

Elevated levels of oestrogen (e.g. during pregnancy and intrauterine life) increase the levels of TBG. These levels are depressed by glucocorticoids, androgens and danazol.

265. ACE

The fetal thyroid is dependent on fetal TSH, independent of the maternal TSH and totally dependent upon the mother for supplies of iodine. TSH secretion in newborns and infants is increased by cold exposure, an effect that is not present in adults. Due to the drop in ambient temperature at birth, the TSH levels in the newborn rise sharply within 30 minutes of delivery and remain so for up to 72 hours before returning to normal.

266. BCE

During pregnancy the glomerular filtration rate increases, leading to a reduction in the tubular absorption of iodide and a doubling of its urinary excretion. This leads to a fall in plasma iodide levels. As a result, the thyroid gland almost triples its iodide trapping from the blood, increasing its size and thyroid hormone production. Also during pregnancy, the raised oestrogen levels cause a rise in TBG levels. The net effect is increased levels of bound and total thyroid hormones, but normal levels of free thyroid hormones.

267. ACDE

The plasma levels of dehydroepiandrosterone sulphate decrease in pregnancy as a consequence of an increased rate of removal, through extensive hydroxylation in the maternal liver and conversion to oestrogen in the placenta.

268. BCD

Alpha-fetoprotein is produced by the yolk sac and the fetal liver. The placenta lacks 16-hydroxylase enzyme necessary to form 16-OH DHAS.

269. BDE

The placenta is the major site of oestrogen production in pregnancy, and it has been shown that the levels of urinary oestrogen do not decrease after bilateral oophorectomy performed as early as 8 weeks gestation. Most of the weight gain in pregnancy occurs during the second and third trimesters.

270. ABDE

The decidua parietalis and the decidua capsularis remain separated during the first trimester, and give the characteristic 'double decidual sign' on ultrasound. They fuse at about 12 weeks gestation.

9

Biochemistry

BIOCHEMISTRY: QUESTIONS

271. During pregnancy there is a rise in the plasma concentration of:
   A. alpha 1-globulin.
   B. albumin.
   C. beta-globulin.
   D. triglycerides.
   E. aspartate aminotransferase.

272. Essential amino acids:
   A. are absorbed from the intestine by active transport.
   B. concentrations in maternal circulation fall during pregnancy.
   C. have higher levels in maternal blood than those in fetal blood.
   D. include phenylalanine.
   E. cross the placenta by simple diffusion.

273. Vitamin B$_{12}$:
   A. serum levels are lower in smokers than in non-smokers.
   B. deficiency leads to megaloblastic anaemia.
   C. supplements are needed in pregnancy.
   D. is absorbed mainly in the stomach, aided by the gastric intrinsic factor.
   E. deficiency anaemia is usually associated with leucopenia.

274. Vitamin E:
   A. is fat-soluble.
   B. is an antioxidant.

C. supplements increase virility in men.

D. deficiency in preterm babies is associated with haemolytic anaemia.

E. supplements potentiate the action of coumarin anti-coagulants.

275. Vitamin B$_{12}$:

A. is fat-soluble.

B. is actively transferred across the placenta.

C. deficiency is common in strict vegetarians (true vegans).

D. is essential for the metabolism of folic acid in humans.

E. in the circulation is mostly attached to a glycoprotein.

276. Vitamin A:

A. is fat-soluble.

B. daily requirement during pregnancy is about 1000 μg.

C. absorption is facilitated by bile salts in the duodenum.

D. deficiency is a common cause of blindness world-wide.

E. is stored in the liver.

277. Thiamine:

A. acts as an antioxidant.

B. is fat-soluble.

C. deficiency may lead to high cardiac output failure.

D. deficiency is associated with heavy alcohol intake.

E. stores in the body are adequate for up to 6 months.

278. Ascorbic acid:

A. is present in high concentrations in the liver.

B. deficiency results in defective collagen formation.

C. excess can lead to the formation of oxalate stones in the urinary tract.

D. is abundantly present in cooked green vegetables.

E. requirements are increased by taking exogenous glucocorticoids.

279. Riboflavin:

    A. is water-soluble.

    B. is exclusively from animal sources.

    C. deficiency can lead to angular stomatitis.

    D. is destroyed by exposure to ultraviolet light.

    E. concentration is higher in the fetus than it is in the mother.

280. Vitamin K:

    A. can reverse the anticoagulant effects of heparin.

    B. is synthesized by bacteria in the colon.

    C. deficiency is the usual cause of haemorrhagic disease of newborn.

    D. is water-soluble.

    E. supplementation is necessary during pregnancy.

281. Vitamin D:

    A. excess can lead to nephrocalcinosis.

    B. is destroyed by ultraviolet light.

    C. increases calcium absorption from the intestine.

    D. is water-soluble.

    E. is hydroxylated in the liver and kidney.

282. Niacin:

    A. deficiency in humans leads to a recognized clinical condition.

    B. is fat-soluble.

    C. is easily destroyed by heat.

    D. is synthesized in the body from tryptophan.

    E. is present in yeast.

283. Vitamin B_6 (pyridoxine):

    A. is water-soluble.

    B. deficiency can lead to epileptiform convulsions.

    C. excess can lead to sensory polyneuropathy.

    D. requirement in pregnancy is 25 mg per day.

    E. deficiency can lead to macrocytic anaemia.

284. Essential amino acids include:

    A. tyrosine.

    B. aspartic acid.

    C. valine.

    D. methionine.

    E. tryptophan.

285. Amino acids that are supplied to the fetus by placental synthesis include:

    A. histidine.

    B. glutamic acid.

    C. valine.

    D. alanine.

    E. leucine.

286. Proteins:

    A. yield 4 calories per gram absorbed.

    B. form hormone receptors in cell membranes.

    C. contain about 50% nitrogen.

    D. turnover in the fetus is higher than that in the mother.

    E. digestion in the stomach is enhanced by a high pH.

287. Vitamin D:

    A. requires fats and bile salts to be efficiently absorbed.

    B. levels in the fetus are higher than those in the mother.

    C. stimulates the absorption of phosphate from the intestine.

    D. crosses the placenta.

    E. is formed by the human placenta.

288. Proteins:

    A. are synthesized in the human body from inorganic sources.

    B. contain amino acids which are always of the L configuration.

    C. are metabolized for energy in preference to carbohydrates.

D. of animal origin have higher nutritional value than those of plant origin.

E. form collagen in connective tissue.

289. The fetal gut:

A. is derived from the mesoderm.

B. absorbs swallowed amniotic fluid.

C. begins to secrete bile by the second trimester.

D. begins to secrete digestive enzymes by the second trimester.

E. does not contain meconium before 28 weeks.

290. Positive nitrogen balance is present during:

A. pregnancy.

B. Cushing's syndrome.

C. pubertal growth.

D. long-term recovery from severe illness.

E. prolonged starvation.

291. Prostaglandins:

A. are metabolized in the lung.

B. contain 18 carbon atoms only.

C. are saturated fatty acids.

D. have a biological half-life of about 30 minutes.

E. maintain the patency of the ductus arteriosus *in utero*.

292. Prostaglandins:

A. $F_{2\alpha}$ stimulate uterine contractions in the non-pregnant uterus.

B. are produced by human red blood cells.

C. E_2 stimulate uterine contractions in the non-pregnant uterus.

D. E_2 contract gut muscle.

E. $F_{2\alpha}$ plasma levels rise during spontaneous labour.

293. Creatine is:

A. synthesized in the liver.

B. converted directly to creatinine.

  C. normally present in the urine of adult men.

  D. normally present in the urine of postnatal women.

  E. synthesized from glycine.

294. Creatinine:

  A. is formed in the kidney.

  B. plasma levels are proportional to the total muscle mass.

  C. plasma levels are raised in renal failure.

  D. plasma levels normally fall during pregnancy.

  E. is excreted mainly by filtration in the kidney.

295. Purines:

  A. include uracil.

  B. are metabolized into uric acid.

  C. are mainly synthesized in the lungs.

  D. enter in the formation of nucleic acids.

  E. are synthesized from amino acids.

296. Uric acid:

  A. is formed by the breakdown of pyrimidines.

  B. in the urine is mainly from renal filtration.

  C. may form renal stones.

  D. production is inhibited by allopurinol.

  E. renal tubular reabsorption is increased in pregnancy.

297. In prolonged starvation there is increased:

  A. plasma free fatty acids.

  B. urinary creatinine.

  C. urinary nitrogen.

  D. plasma cortisol levels.

  E. insulin secretion.

298. Glycogen synthesis is increased by:

  A. glucose.

  B. insulin.

C. glucagon.

D. adrenaline.

E. starvation.

299. **Glycolysis:**

A. requires oxygen.

B. is energy-dependent.

C. converts glucose to carbon dioxide and water.

D. of a molecule of glucose leads to a net gain of two molecules of ATP.

E. in the liver is inhibited by insulin.

300. **The Krebs (citric acid) cycle:**

A. can function under anaerobic conditions.

B. occurs inside the mitochondria.

C. is the common pathway for oxidation of carbohydrate and fat.

D. involves the release of four carbon atoms at each turn of the cycle.

E. is entered only through acetyl coenzyme A (CoA).

301. **In aerobic glycolysis:**

A. glucose is converted to lactate.

B. one molecule of glucose produces 38 molecules of ATP.

C. carbon dioxide and water are produced.

D. one molecule of NADH generates two molecules of ATP.

E. oxidative phosphorylation occurs in the Krebs cycle.

302. **Glucogenic amino acids include:**

A. alanine.

B. isoleucine.

C. tyrosine.

D. proline.

E. valine.

303. In relation to fat metabolism:

   A. carnitine inhibits fat oxidation.

   B. the catabolism of one molecule of a 6-carbon atom fatty acid through the Krebs cycle yields 44 molecules ATP.

   C. activation of fatty acids occurs exclusively in the mitochondria.

   D. beta-oxidation of fatty acids is inhibited by high glucose blood level.

   E. free fatty acids in the circulation are bound to albumin.

304. Acetone is:

   A. formed in the liver.

   B. excreted in expired air.

   C. a ketone body.

   D. formed by oxidation of acetoacetic acid.

   E. excreted in the urine.

305. Cholesterol:

   A. is the precursor of progesterone.

   B. is synthesized in the liver.

   C. concentration in the plasma is increased by oestrogen.

   D. is synthesized from acetate.

   E. plasma levels rise during the third trimester of normal pregnancy.

306. Amino acid detoxification through the urea cycle:

   A. occurs mainly in the kidney.

   B. occurs exclusively in the mitochondria.

   C. is energy-dependent.

   D. involves the formation of citrulline from ornithine and carbamoyl phosphate.

   E. yields urea and ornithine.

307. With regard to carbohydrate metabolism:

   A. the transport of fructose from the intestines to the blood stream is energy-dependent.

    B. galactose is composed of glucose and lactose.

    C. there is increased plasma insulin level during the second half of pregnancy.

    D. oestrogens increase fasting blood glucose level.

    E. carbohydrate excess leads to ketosis.

308. Enzymes are:

    A. proteins.

    B. activated by heat.

    C. affected by changes in pH.

    D. made more soluble by the addition of organic solvents.

    E. present only in the mitochondria.

309. Pyrimidines:

    A. are catabolized to CO_2 and H_2O.

    B. include thymine.

    C. are synthesized in the liver.

    D. combine with ribose to form nucleosides.

    E. are components of amino acids.

310. Folic acid:

    A. is water-soluble.

    B. is absorbed mainly in the jejunum.

    C. supplements are given with methotrexate therapy to reduce side-effects.

    D. deficiency leads to macrocytic anaemia.

    E. supplements reduce the chance of recurrence of neural tube defect.

▌ BIOCHEMISTRY: ANSWERS

271. ACD

Albumin concentration falls during normal pregnancy; a steep fall in the first trimester is followed by a slower fall during the second and third trimesters. Aspartate aminotransferase levels remain unchanged in normal pregnancy. Pathological conditions involving the liver, such as pre-eclampsia, can lead to a rise in aspartate aminotransferase and a further fall in albumin.

272. ABD

Essential amino acids are transferred across the placenta to the fetus by active transport. Consequently, their levels in the fetal blood are far higher than they are in the maternal circulation.

273. ABE

The cyanide content of the tobacco smoke is detoxified by a mechanism which depletes the store of vitamin B_{12}, hence its lower levels in smokers. Vitamin B_{12} is stored in the liver where there may be up to 3 years supply. Therefore, supplements are not normally needed in pregnancy. It is absorbed mainly in the lower ileum, aided by the gastric intrinsic factor.

274. ABDE

Although vitamin E deficiency has been shown to cause testicular degeneration, abortion and fetal death in animals, there is no scientific evidence that supplements increase virility or are useful in the treatment of infertility or recurrent abortion in humans. Vitamin E deficiency in preterm babies (especially those weighing less than 1.5 kg) is associated with haemolytic anaemia.

275. BCDE

Vitamin B_{12} is water-soluble. Its levels in the umbilical cord blood are higher than in normal adults due to its active placental transfer. It is obtained mainly from animal foodstuffs and vegetables alone are an inadequate source.

276. ABCDE

Vitamin A (retinol) is essential for maintenance of epithelial tissue, including the corneal epithelium. It is also an essential component of the pigmented rhodopsin (in the retina) which is responsible for night vision. The World Health Organization (WHO) estimates that 250 000 children become blind every year from keratomalacia secondary to vitamin A deficiency.

277. CD

Thiamine (vitamin B$_1$) is water-soluble and is essential for oxidative decarboxylation of pyruvate to acetyl coenzyme A. When deficient, there is accumulation of pyruvic and lactic acids which leads to vasodilatation and increases cardiac output. Deficiency can also lead to neurological manifestations as the cells cannot utilize glucose aerobically and the nervous system depends entirely on glucose for its energy requirements. The body contains only 30 mg thiamine, 30 times the adult daily requirement.

278. BCE

Ascorbic acid (vitamin C) is present in high concentration in the eye and the adrenal cortex. Stress, corticotrophin secretion and exogenous glucocorticoids lead to a loss of ascorbic acid from the adrenal cortex and increase the daily requirements. Ascorbic acid is very soluble in water and easily destroyed by heat. For these reasons cooking reduces or even eliminates it from the diet.

279. ACDE

Animal sources (e.g. liver, kidney) as well as plant sources (e.g. wheat, bran, mushrooms) are rich in riboflavin (vitamin B$_2$). Water-soluble vitamins (such as riboflavin) cross the placenta by active mechanisms which result in higher concentrations in the fetus.

280. BC

Vitamin K is fat-soluble. As it is synthesized by colonic bacteria, no external supplements are necessary. An exception is in newborn babies whose colons have not yet been colonized by bacteria. It is essential for carboxylation of clotting factors II, VII, IX and X in the liver. Carboxylation of the glutamyl residues in these factors increases their negative charges and allows them to bind to phospholipid surfaces particularly on the platelet. Warfarin inhibits this carboxylation and vitamin K is used to reverse the anticoagulant effects of warfarin. Heparin, on the other hand, produces its anticoagulant action by potentiating the antithrombin III activity. Protamine sulphate is used to reverse the action of heparin.

281. ACE

Vitamin D (cholecalciferol) is fat-soluble. It is formed in the skin by the action of ultraviolet light on 7-dehydrocholesterol. In the liver it is converted to 25-hydroxycholecalciferol, which is further hydroxylated in the kidney, mainly to 1,25-dihydroxycholecalciferol.

282. ADE

Niacin (a member of the vitamin B group) is water-soluble and resistant to heat. Its deficiency leads to pellagra (dermatitis, diarrhoea, stomatitis, glossitis, dementia).

283. ABC

Pyridoxine requirement in pregnancy is 2.5 mg/day. Its deficiency leads to microcytic anaemia, gastrointestinal disturbance, and neuritis. It also leads to convulsions; an epidemic of convulsions in infants in the USA in the 1950s was traced to a milk formula deficient in pyridoxine because of a manufacturing error.

284. CDE

Essential amino acids are those not synthesized in the body in an adequate amount to fulfil normal requirements. They include threonine, lysine, methionine, tryptophan, valine, phenylalanine, leucine and isoleucine. Histidine and arginine are sometimes included in this list and although they are required for normal growth they are not 'essential' in the strict sense of the definition.

285. BD

The placenta synthesizes acidic non-essential amino acids (e.g. glutamic acid) and neutral straight-chain amino acids (e.g. alanine), and these amino acids are not absorbed from the maternal blood. On the other hand, the essential neutral branched-chain amino acids (e.g. valine and leucine) and basic amino acids (histidine) are transferred across the placenta from the mother to the fetus by active transport.

286. BD

Each gram of protein yields 4 kilocalories (1 kcal = 1000 calories). Proteins on average contain 16% nitrogen and 84% carbon, hydrogen and sulphur. In the stomach the parietal cells secrete HCl, leading to a low pH. This causes the hydrolysis of pepsinogen (secreted from the chief cells) into pepsin, which is a proteolytic enzyme.

287. ACDE

Fetal levels of vitamin D are substantially lower than those in the mother and rise rapidly in the first 2 days postpartum.

288. BDE

Only plants and micro-organisms are able to synthesize proteins from inorganic sources. Higher organisms and animals (including humans) must be supplied with proteins exogenously. Carbohydrates are metabolized for energy in preference to proteins.

289. BCD

The fetal gut differentiates from the endoderm. As early as 16 weeks meconium is present in the fetal gut and consists of desquamated intestinal cells, intestinal juices and squamous cells.

290. ACD

Nitrogen balance is the balance between the intake of nitrogenous compounds (mainly as proteins) and their excretion (mainly in the urine, as excretion in the faeces, sweat and menstrual blood is normally minimal). When the amount of urinary nitrogen is equal to the amount of nitrogen in the protein in the diet, the individual is said to be in nitrogen balance. Conditions in which there is formation of new tissues (pregnancy, growth) or tissue repair (recovery from illness) lead to positive balance. Conditions in which there is diminished intake (starvation), increased tissue breakdown (illness, immobilization) or increased secretion of catabolic hormones (Cushing's syndrome) lead to negative balance.

291. AE

Prostaglandins are a group of 20-carbon polyunsaturated fatty acids containing a cyclopentane ring. They are also called eicosanoids, reflecting their origin from the 20-carbon (eicosa-) arachidonic acid. The different groups of prostaglandins (e.g. E, F) are classified according to the configuration of the cyclopentane ring. For each group a subscript numeral denotes the degree of unsaturation (double bonds) in the side chain. They have a relatively short half-life (e.g. prostacyclin: 3 minutes; thromboxane: 30 seconds) and usually exert their biological action at the site of release.

292. ADE

Prostaglandins $F_{2\alpha}$ stimulate myometrial contractions in the pregnant and the non-pregnant uterus. Prostaglandins E_2, on the other hand, relax the non-pregnant uterus but stimulate myometrial contractions during pregnancy. All mammalian cells except the red blood cells produce prostaglandins. The plasma levels of prostaglandins $F_{2\alpha}$ do not vary significantly throughout pregnancy, but are elevated during spontaneous labour.

293. ADE

Creatine is synthesized in the liver from glycine, methionine and arginine. In the skeletal muscles it is phosphorylated to form phosphorylcreatine, which acts as an important energy store. Creatinine is formed from phosphorylcreatine, and not directly from creatine. Creatinuria occurs normally in children, pregnant, and postnatal women but not in adult men. It is also present when there is extensive muscle breakdown (e.g. starvation, thyrotoxicosis).

294. BCDE

Creatinine is formed in muscle from phosphorylcreatine. It is excreted in the urine mainly by filtration, though a small amount is secreted.

295. BDE

The principal physiologically important purines are: adenine, guanine, hypoxanthine and xanthine. Uracil is a pyrimidine. Purines are mainly synthesized in the liver and enter in the formation of nucleic acids, coenzymes and related substances such as ATP.

296. CDE

Uric acid is formed by the breakdown of purines. It is filtered, reabsorbed and secreted in the kidney. Normally, 98% of the filtered uric acid is reabsorbed and the remaining 2% makes up about 20% of the amount excreted in the urine. The remaining 80% comes from tubular secretion. During pregnancy, the clearance of uric acid is increased, but this is balanced by increased tubular reabsorption. The net result is that the plasma levels of uric acid do not change significantly during pregnancy.

297. ACD

In prolonged starvation there is low urinary creatinine and diminished insulin secretion.

298. AB

Glucagon, adrenaline and low plasma glucose levels (as in starvation) lead to increased glycogen breakdown (glycogenolysis).

299. BD

Glycolysis involves phosphorylation of glucose, which is an energy-dependent step. For each molecule of glucose two molecules of ATP are needed and four molecules are yielded, leading to a net production of two ATP molecules. Glucose is converted to pyruvate and lactate in an oxygen-independent series of reactions. Insulin stimulates glucokinase (a major glycolytic enzyme in the liver).

300. BC

The Krebs cycle requires oxygen and does not function under anaerobic conditions. For each turn of the cycle four pairs of carbon atoms are released in the form of nicotinamide adenine dinucleotide (NADH). Although major entry into the cycle is through acetyl CoA, pyruvate can enter also by taking up CO_2 to form oxaloacetate, and some amino acids can be converted to citric acid cycle intermediates by deamination.

301. BC

The formation of lactate from glucose occurs in the absence of oxygen (anaerobic glycolysis). Aerobically, one molecule of NADH generates three ATP molecules. During aerobic glycolysis hydrogen is produced (in the form of NADH) in the Krebs cycle. NADH, following that, undergoes oxidative phosphorylation in the respiratory chain (flavoprotein-cytochrome system).

302. ADE

Glucogenic amino acids are those giving rise to compounds that can readily be converted to glucose. They include alanine, arginine, aspartic acid, cysteine, glutamic acid, glycine, histidine, proline, serine, threonine and valine. Ketogenic amino acids are those that can be converted to the ketone body acetoacetate and include leucine, isoleucine, phenylalanine and tyrosine.

303. BD

Fatty acid oxidation begins with activation of the fatty acid and this reaction occurs both inside and outside the mitochondria. Active long-chain fatty acids formed outside the mitochondria must be linked to carnitine (a derivative of lysine) to cross the mitochondrial membrane. Carnitine, therefore, stimulates fat oxidation.

304. ABCE

In conditions leading to deficient intracellular glucose supply (such as starvation and diabetes mellitus) there is increased lipolysis to cope with the energy needs of the tissues. Lipolysis yields acetyl CoA which, under normal conditions, enters the citric acid cycle. With increased lipolysis there is more acetyl CoA produced than can enter the citric acid cycle. This excess acetyl CoA is converted in the liver to acetoacetic acid, which is either reduced to beta hydroxybutyric acid or decarboxylated to acetone.

305. ABDE

Cholesterol is the precursor of all steroid hormones. The plasma cholesterol level is decreased by oestrogen, which also lowers the low density lipoproteins (LDL) and increases the high density lipoproteins (HDL).

306. CDE

The liver is the major site for amino acid detoxification. The first few reactions of the urea cycle occur in the mitochondria, while the latter parts of the cycle take place in the cytoplasm.

307. C

The intestinal transport of glucose and galactose is an energy-dependent active process, while the transport of fructose is passive. Lactose is composed of glucose and galactose. Oestrogens lower fasting blood glucose level; they increase both insulin and glucagon production by the pancreas, but with a rise in the insulin : glucagon ratio. Carbohydrate deprivation (and not excess) leads to ketosis as fatty acids are metabolized for energy and ketone bodies are produced.

308. AC

The three-dimensional configuration of an enzyme is crucial to its activity and maintained by hydrogen bonds. These bonds are rather weak and readily disrupted by heat. Heating an enzyme, therefore, usually results in loss of activity. Enzyme solubility is reduced by the addition of organic solvents. Enzymes are present in all cell organelles (e.g. nucleus, cytosol, microsomes, mitochondria).

309. BCD

Pyrimidines include cytosine, uracil and thymine. They are synthesized from amino acids and catabolized to CO_2 and NH_3.

310. ABDE

Methotrexate is an antimetabolite which binds competitively to the enzyme dihydrofolate reductase. This enzyme is necessary in folate metabolism to produce tetrahydrofolates, which are essential for both purine and pyrimidine biosynthesis. This biochemical blockade can be bypassed by giving folinic acid (exogenous tetrahydrofolates) and not folic acid.

10

Pharmacology

PHARMACOLOGY: QUESTIONS

311. Drugs which can cause hirsutism include:

    A. methyl-testosterone.

    B. phenytoin.

    C. cyproterone acetate.

    D. diazoxide.

    E. danazol.

312. Stimulation of beta-adrenergic receptors is caused by:

    A. ritodrine.

    B. pentolinium.

    C. terbutaline.

    D. metaraminol.

    E. nifedipine.

313. Parasympathomimetic drugs include:

    A. probanthine.

    B. pilocarpine.

    C. scopolamine.

    D. muscarine.

    E. atropine.

314. Drugs that cross the placenta include:

    A. heparin.

    B. warfarin.

    C. insulin.

    D. methyldopa.

    E. penicillin.

315. Recognized side-effects of clomiphene citrate include:

    A. postural hypotension.

    B. blurring of vision.

    C. alopecia.

    D. hot flushes.

    E. nausea.

316. Drugs not effective if taken orally include:

    A. progesterone.

    B. insulin.

    C. heparin.

    D. human chorionic gonadotrophin.

    E. ergometrine.

317. Recognized side-effects of the combined oral contraceptive pill include increased incidence of:

    A. ovarian cancer.

    B. endometrial cancer.

    C. pelvic inflammatory disease.

    D. venous thrombosis.

    E. ectopic pregnancy.

318. The activity of hepatic enzymes is increased by the administration of:

    A. phenytoin.

    B. cimetidine.

    C. heparin.

    D. rifampicin.

    E. griseofulvin.

319. Beta-adrenoceptor blockers:

    A. are contraindicated during pregnancy.

    B. are contraindicated during breast feeding.

    C. stimulate uterine contractions.

    D. cause peripheral vasoconstriction.

    E. inhibit renin release from the kidney.

320. The following drugs are contraindicated during breast feeding:

    A. warfarin.

    B. methyldopa.

    C. penicillin.

    D. metronidazole.

    E. carbamazepine.

321. Side-effects of frusemide include:

    A. acidosis.

    B. hyperglycaemia.

    C. hyperkalaemia.

    D. pancreatitis.

    E. hyperlipidaemia.

322. Spironolactone:

    A. can cause hirsutism.

    B. potentiates digitalis toxicity.

    C. is an aldosterone antagonist.

    D. has strong progestogenic activity.

    E. causes potassium depletion.

323. Methyldopa:

    A. acts mainly on the peripheral alpha-adrenergic receptors.

    B. can cause a positive direct antiglobulin (Coombs') test.

    C. is a fast-acting hypotensive agent.

    D. can cause depression.

    E. can cause haemolytic anaemia.

324. The following are hypotensive agents used in pregnancy:

    A. nifedipine.

    B. hydralazine.

C. captopril.

D. labetalol.

E. chlorothiazide.

325. The main mechanism of action of:

A. hydralazine is alpha-adrenergic receptor blocking.

B. nifedipine is calcium-entry blocking.

C. labetalol is beta-adrenergic receptor blocking.

D. verapamil is direct arterial vasodilatation.

E. methyldopa is alpha-adrenergic receptor blocking.

326. Benzylpenicillin:

A. crosses the placenta.

B. is active against beta-haemolytic streptococcus.

C. must be administered parenterally.

D. inhibits bacterial cell wall synthesis.

E. can lead to delayed hypersensitivity reactions.

327. Tetracyclines:

A. are bactericidal.

B. are active against chlamydial infections.

C. can cause impaired fetal bone growth.

D. are associated with acute fatty liver in pregnancy.

E. can be administered orally.

328. Antibiotics effective against *Staphylococcus aureus* include:

A. cloxacillin.

B. cephalosporins.

C. fucidin.

D. clindamycin.

E. gentamicin.

329. Bactericidal antibiotics include:

A. ampicillin.

B. doxicycline.

C. trimethoprim.

D. streptomycin.

E. cefuroxime.

330. The following drugs potentiate the anticoagulant effect of warfarin:

A. rifampicin.

B. carbamazepine.

C. ampicillin.

D. cimetidine.

E. sulphonamides.

331. The following are orally active oestrogens:

A. mestranol.

B. megestrol acetate.

C. oestradiol valerate.

D. ethinyl oestradiol.

E. oestrogen benzoate.

332. The combined oral contraceptive pill leads to a decrease in:

A. glucose tolerance.

B. antithrombin III plasma concentration.

C. thyroid-binding globulin plasma concentration.

D. triglycerides plasma concentration.

E. the incidence of liver adenoma.

333. The contraceptive efficacy of the combined pill can be reduced if concurrently taken with:

A. sodium valproate.

B. ampicillin.

C. cyproterone acetate.

D. primidone.

E. vitamin K.

334. Warfarin:

A. crosses the placenta.

B. is teratogenic.

C. is albumin-bound.

D. is the anticoagulant drug of choice in pregnant women with prosthetic heart valves.

E. is only active *in vivo*.

335. Recognized side-effects of heparin include:

A. teratogenicity if used in the first trimester.

B. thrombocytopaenia.

C. osteoporosis.

D. hypersensitivity reactions.

E. haemorrhage.

336. Postmenopausal oestrogen hormone replacement therapy leads to an increase in:

A. the incidence of venous thrombosis.

B. high-density lipoprotein cholesterol.

C. low-density lipoprotein cholesterol.

D. triglycerides.

E. the incidence of stroke.

337. Morphine:

A. must be administered parenterally in order to have a therapeutic effect.

B. is an opioid receptor agonist.

C. can cause bronchoconstriction.

D. inhibits the release of antidiuretic hormone.

E. inhibits gut motility.

338. Pethidine:

A. has a shorter half-life than naloxone.

B. induced analgesic effects are not reversed by naloxone.

C. does not cross the placenta.

D. has a more rapid onset than heroin.

E. is contraindicated in asthmatic women in labour.

339. Curare:
- A. crosses the placenta.
- B. is excreted by the kidney.
- C. may be potentiated by gentamicin.
- D. exerts its effect at the level of the acetylcholine receptor.
- E. can cause hypotension due to its direct effect on the arterial wall smooth muscles.

340. Halothane:
- A. causes uterine relaxation.
- B. is hepatotoxic.
- C. causes reactive hypertension.
- D. can cause myocardial depression.
- E. crosses the placenta.

341. Suxamethonium:
- A. is a 'non-depolarizing' muscle relaxant.
- B. has rapid action.
- C. causes muscle fasciculation.
- D. increases intraocular pressure.
- E. is a uterine relaxant.

342. The use of ritodrine in preterm labour can lead to a rise in:
- A. maternal heart rate.
- B. fetal heart rate.
- C. serum glucose.
- D. serum potassium.
- E. blood pressure.

343. Side-effects of oxytocin include:
- A. fetal distress.
- B. hypernatraemia.
- C. amniotic fluid embolism.
- D. uterine rupture.
- E. hyperprolactinaemia.

344. Drugs which affect the uterus include:

    A. magnesium sulphate.

    B. indomethacin.

    C. aminophylline.

    D. ethanol.

    E. nifedipine.

345. Bromocriptine:

    A. is a dopamine agonist.

    B. is contraindicated in cases of pituitary adenoma.

    C. action is potentiated by tricyclic antidepressants.

    D. is used as an antihypertensive agent.

    E. is used for suppression of lactation.

346. Drugs which are teratogenic in the human include:

    A. bromocriptine.

    B. methyldopa.

    C. metronidazole.

    D. carbamazepine.

    E. diethylstilboestrol.

347. Smoking during pregnancy is associated with increased incidence of:

    A. preterm labour.

    B. intrauterine growth retardation

    C. pre-eclampsia.

    D. placental abruption.

    E. iron deficiency anaemia.

348. Side-effects of phenothiazines include:

    A. diarrhoea.

    B. hyperprolactinaemia.

    C. hyperthermia.

    D. dystonia.

    E. blurring of vision.

349. The following drugs are monoamine oxidase inhibitors:

    A. imipramine.

    B. phenelzine.

    C. pericyazine.

    D. iproniazid.

    E. pimozide.

350. Ergometrine:

    A. is an oxytocic.

    B. is used for induction of labour.

    C. when given intramuscularly, acts within 2 minutes.

    D. can cause vomiting.

    E. may cause an acute rise in blood pressure.

351. The following drugs are alkylating agents:

    A. mercaptopurine.

    B. cyclophosphamide.

    C. methotrexate.

    D. chlorambucil.

    E. vinblastine.

352. The following drugs could be administered orally in the treatment of cancer:

    A. medroxyprogesterone acetate.

    B. methotrexate.

    C. cisplatinum.

    D. cyclophosphamide.

    E. chlorambucil.

353. Methotrexate:

    A. is used in the treatment of ectopic pregnancy.

    B. is excreted in the urine.

    C. can lead to throat ulceration.

    D. is used in the treatment of advanced carcinoma of the cervix.

    E. leads to ovarian failure.

354. Cyclophosphamide:

    A. is excreted mainly in the urine.

    B. can lead to haematuria.

    C. can cause alopecia.

    D. may lead to ovarian failure.

    E. is used in the treatment of rheumatoid arthritis.

355. Recognized side-effects of bleomycin include:

    A. pulmonary fibrosis.

    B. severe bone marrow suppression.

    C. alopecia.

    D. skin pigmentation.

    E. mucositis.

░ PHARMACOLOGY: ANSWERS

311. ABDE

Cyproterone acetate is an anti-androgen used in the treatment of hirsutism. It also has progestational activity and is a component of some combined oral contraceptive pills (e.g. Dianette).

312. AC

Pentolinium is a ganglion-blocking agent, metaraminol is an alpha-receptor agonist, and nifedipine is a calcium-channel blocking agent. Beta-agonists cause reduction in uterine contractions (β_2 receptor action) and are used to suppress preterm labour. Nifedipine may also be used, but acts through a different mechanism.

313. BD

Probanthine, scopolamine and atropine are parasympatholytics. Pilocarpine and muscarine are anticholinesterase drugs and thus act as parasympathomimetics.

314. BDE

Because of their high molecular weight, heparin and insulin do not cross the placenta.

315. BCDE

Clomiphene citrate (widely used for induction of ovulation) has both oestrogenic and antioestrogenic activities. The oestrogenic action may lead to nausea and blurring of vision (through its effect on the cornea), while the antioestrogenic action may lead to alopecia and hot flushes.

316. ABCD

Although ergometrine is usually administered parenterally, there is actually an oral preparation. All the other drugs in the question have to be administered parenterally to have an effect.

317. D

The incidence of ovarian and endometrial cancers, pelvic inflammatory disease, and ectopic pregnancy is actually decreased in the users of the combined oral contraceptive pill.

318. ADE

These 'enzyme inducers' will lead to accelerated elimination and reduced efficacy of drugs that are metabolized by the same enzymes. This is the reason why women who are on anticonvulsants such as phenytoin and carbamazepine (enzyme inducers) have a higher rate of failure when taking the combined oral contraceptive pill (which is metabolized in the liver).

319. DE

Beta-blockers are used for treatment of hypertension during pregnancy and are also considered safe during breast feeding. Although beta-agonists inhibit uterine contractions, there is no evidence that beta-blockers have any effect on uterine musculature.

320. ALL ARE FALSE

All these drugs may be safely prescribed during breast feeding. It is also important to reassure the breast-feeding mother that the drugs will not adversely affect the baby as this may increase her compliance with the treatment.

321. BDE

Frusemide is a potent 'loop diuretic' which acts by inhibiting sodium and potassium reabsorption in the ascending loop of Henle. It can cause hypokalaemia and hypochloraemic alkalosis.

322. BC

Spironolactone is a potassium-sparing diuretic and can lead to hyperkalaemia, which may potentiate digitalis toxicity. Spironolactone also has some antiandrogen effect and is used in the treatment of hirsutism.

323. BDE

Methyldopa is an alpha$_2$ agonist widely used in the treatment of hypertension during pregnancy. It acts, through its metabolite alpha-methylnoradrenaline, on the central alpha$_2$ receptors in the brain to reduce the sympathetic outflow. Methyldopa is slow-acting and, therefore, not suitable for emergency treatment of hypertension when a more rapid hypotensive effect is required.

324. ABD

Captopril (an angiotensin-converting enzyme inhibitor) and chlorothiazide (a thiazide diuretic) are hypotensive agents but are not used during pregnancy.

325. BC

Hydralazine causes direct arterial vasodilatation, verapamil is a calcium-channel blocking agent, and methyldopa is a centrally acting $alpha_2$-receptor agonist. Labetalol also has some alpha-adrenergic blocking action.

326. ABCDE

Benzylpenicillin (and the penicillins in general) cross the placenta and achieve fetal levels reaching about 70% of those in the mother. They are, therefore, used in cases of fetal infection such as congenital syphilis.

327. BCDE

Tetracyclines are broad-spectrum bacteriostatic antibiotics. They bind to calcium and, if taken antenatally or during childhood, can impair bone growth and lead to teeth discoloration. Before these facts were discovered tetracyclines were used during pregnancy and were found to be associated with the development of acute fatty liver.

328. ABCDE

Staphylococcus aureus is a Gram-positive organism which causes wound infection and abscesses. Penicillinase-producing *S. aureus* (which is the main type isolated in hospital) is resistant to penicillin and ampicillin.

329. ACDE

Doxicycline is bacteriostatic. Ampicillin and cefuroxime inhibit bacterial cell wall synthesis, trimethoprim inhibits the conversion of folate into tetrahydrofolate, and streptomycin acts at the level of the ribosome.

330. CDE

Rifampicin, carbamazepine, phenytoin, griseofulvin and barbiturates are enzyme inducers and reduce the anticoagulant effect of warfarin. Cimetidine and sulphonamides are enzyme inhibitors and potentiate the action of warfarin. Ampicillin is a broad-spectrum antibiotic which affects the gut flora and interferes with vitamin K synthesis and enhances warfarin activity.

331. ACD

Mestranol is the oestrogen commonly used in the older oral contraceptive pills and ethinyl oestradiol is the one most widely used in current pills. Oestradiol valerate is used in hormone replacement therapy and is converted to oestrone during absorption. Oestrogen benzoate is not active orally and megestrol is a derivative of 17α-hydroxyprogesterone.

332. AB

The incidence of liver adenoma and the plasma concentration of thyroid-binding globulin and triglycerides increase in women taking the combined oral contraceptive pill.

333. BD

Sodium valproate is one of the few antiepileptic drugs that do not interfere with the action of the pill. Most of the other commonly used antiepileptics (such as carbamazepine and phenytoin) are enzyme inducers and can lead to pill failure. Primidone is also an enzyme inducer. Ampicillin interferes with the enterohepatic circulation of the pill. Cyproterone acetate is an antiandrogen and is actually a constituent of some contraceptive pills (e.g. Dianette).

334. ABCDE

Warfarin (a coumarin oral anticoagulant) is teratogenic; if taken during the first trimester it can lead to nasal hypoplasia and chondrodysplasia punctata. Its use later on in pregnancy is also associated with CNS abnormalities. However, it is the anticoagulant of choice in pregnant women with prosthetic heart valves. These women are at a high risk of developing thromboembolic problems and heparin is not as effective as warfarin in preventing these problems.

335. BCDE

Heparin does not cross the placenta and, therefore, is not teratogenic. However, this is not to say that it cannot affect the fetus adversely; if given in large doses it can lead to placental haemorrhage.

336. BD

Postmenopausal oestrogen hormone replacement therapy (HRT) leads to an increase in high-density lipoprotein cholesterol (HDL) and triglycerides and a decrease in low-density lipoprotein cholesterol (LDL). HDL is considered protective against cardiovascular disease (coronary artery disease and stroke) while LDL increases the risk. Indeed, there is epidemiological evidence to suggest that oestrogen HRT reduces the risk of cardiovascular disease. There is no evidence that HRT increases the risk of either venous or arterial thrombosis.

337. BCE

Morphine is active orally as well as parenterally, e.g. oral morphine is usually used for pain relief in cancer patients. Such long-term use is often associated with constipation due to the effect of morphine on gut motility. Morphine stimulates the release of antidiuretic hormone as well as that of histamine (thus causing bronchoconstriction).

338. D

Pethidine (a synthetic opioid agonist) crosses the placenta and, when administered during labour, can lead to neonatal respiratory depression. Naloxone (an opioid antagonist) reverses all the effects of pethidine, including its analgesic action. Naloxone has a shorter half-life than pethidine.

339. BCD

Curare is a muscle relaxant and does not cross the placenta because of its polarity. It causes histamine release, which accounts for its hypotensive effect.

340. ABDE

Halothane is a widely used agent for maintenance of general anaesthesia. It causes hypotension and, on repeated exposure, can lead to liver damage.

341. BCD

Suxamethonium is a muscle relaxant acting on the neuromuscular junction like acetylcholine, but leading to prolonged depolarization. The muscle relaxation is preceded by muscle fasciculation and a sharp rise in plasma potassium and creatine phosphokinase.

342. ABC

Ritodrine and other beta-adrenergic receptor agonists lead to hypotension (through peripheral vasodilatation) and a fall in serum potassium (due to a shift of potassium ions into the cellular compartment).

343. ACD

Oxytocin has about 5% of the antidiuretic effect of the hormone vasopressin and, in large doses, can lead to water intoxication and hyponatraemia. This is more likely if the drug is administered with large amounts of fluid.

344. ABCDE

All these drugs act as tocolytics inhibiting uterine contractions.

345. AE

Bromocriptine is a dopamine agonist used in the treatment of hyperprolactinaemia. It is the drug of choice whether the hyperprolactinaemia is idiopathic or secondary to a pituitary adenoma. Its main side-effect is hypotension, but it is not used as an antihypertensive agent. Tricyclic antidepressants can cause hyperprolactinaemia.

346. DE

Although very large doses of metronidazole are teratogenic in rodents, there is no evidence that it is teratogenic in the human. Carbamazepine and all other commonly used anticonvulsant agents appear to be teratogenic, with a 5–10% incidence of fetal abnormalities. In fact, epilepsy itself seems to be associated with a higher incidence of fetal abnormalities, irrespective of drug treatment. Diethylstilboestrol (DES) leads to a wide spectrum of genital abnormalities in the fetus and is associated with vaginal adenosis and adenocarcinoma of the vagina in the female offspring.

347. ABD

Smokers have a reduced likelihood of developing pre-eclampsia during pregnancy but if they do, they usually have a worse outcome than non-smokers.

348. BDE

Phenothiazines have anticholinergic effects and lead to constipation and difficulty with micturition. Their dopamine receptor blocking action is responsible for the hyperprolactinaemia and extrapyramidal effects such as dystonia. They can also cause hypothermia, weight gain and cholestatic jaundice.

349. BD

Imipramine is a tricyclic antidepressant, pericyazine is a phenothiazine and pimozide is a butyrophenone.

350. ADE

Ergometrine is an oxytocic agent which produces a prolonged tonic uterine contraction with superimposed rapid clonic contractions. It is not used antenatally, but widely used postnatally for the prevention and treatment of postpartum haemorrhage. Given intramuscularly, it takes about 7 minutes to act. This is the reason why it is usually combined with syntocinon (as syntometrine) because intramuscular syntocinon has a more rapid onset.

351. BD

Mercaptopurine is a purine analogue antimetabolite, methotrexate is an antifolic acid, and vinblastine is a vinca alkaloid.

352. ABDE

Cisplatinum is administered intravenously. Medroxyprogesterone acetate is used in the treatment of endometrial carcinoma.

353. ABCD

Methotrexate is used extensively in the treatment of trophoblastic disease and does not lead to ovarian failure. It is also used in the treatment of ectopic pregnancy by systemic administration or by direct injection into the ectopic sac.

354. BCDE

Cyclophosphamide is excreted mostly in the faeces, but about 25% is excreted in the urine and may lead to haemorrhagic cystitis and haematuria. Because of its immunosuppressive action it is used in the treatment of rheumatoid arthritis.

355. ACDE

Bleomycin is relatively free of bone marrow toxicity and its major side-effect is pulmonary fibrosis, which can be quite severe in some cases.

11

Microbiology

MICROBIOLOGY: QUESTIONS

356. Bacteria:

    A. are prokaryotic.

    B. replicate by mitosis.

    C. contain single-stranded deoxyribonucleic acid.

    D. are divided into Gram-positive and Gram-negative according to the staining of the nucleus.

    E. can be seen with the light microscope.

357. The following are Gram-positive bacteria:

    A. *Streptococcus haemolyticus.*

    B. *Neisseria gonorrhoeae.*

    C. *Escherichia coli.*

    D. *Treponema pallidum.*

    E. *Mycobacterium tuberculosis.*

358. Rickettsiae are the causative organisms of:

    A. typhus.

    B. spotted fever.

    C. trench fever.

    D. enteric fever.

    E. scarlet fever.

359. *Staphylococcus aureus:*

    A. produces the enzyme coagulase.

    B. produces exotoxins.

    C. is responsible for erysipelas.

    D. is usually sensitive to ampicillin.

    E. can cause osteomyelitis.

360. **Beta-haemolytic streptococci can cause:**

    A. puerperal sepsis.

    B. neonatal septicaemia.

    C. infective endocarditis.

    D. necrotizing fasciitis.

    E. quinsy.

361. *Corynebacterium diphtheriae:*

    A. is Gram-negative.

    B. infection can lead to myocarditis.

    C. acute infection is diagnosed by Schick's test.

    D. produce toxins.

    E. grows on tellurite medium.

362. *Listeria monocytogenes:*

    A. is motile.

    B. produces haemolysins.

    C. is carried normally in the gut of healthy non-infected individuals.

    D. can be found in soil.

    E. is destroyed by freezing.

363. **Listeriosis:**

    A. can be diagnosed by blood culture.

    B. occurs exclusively in the third trimester.

    C. causes intrauterine death.

    D. can be treated with ampicillin.

    E. has a predilection for immunocompromised individuals.

364. **Meningitis can be caused by:**

    A. herpes virus.

    B. *Listeria monocytogenes.*

    C. *Streptococcus pneumoniae.*

    D. *Neisseria meningitidis.*

    E. *Staphylococcus aureus.*

365. The causative organism of:

    A. condyloma lata is human papilloma virus.

    B. acquired immune deficiency syndrome (AIDS) is a retrovirus.

    C. chancroid is *Haemophilus ducreyoi.*

    D. lymphogranuloma venereum is *Calymmatobacterium granulomatis.*

    E. granuloma inguinale is *Chlamydia trachomatis.*

366. The following factors predispose to vaginal infection with *Candida albicans:*

    A. pregnancy.

    B. the use of broad-spectrum antibiotics.

    C. diabetes mellitus.

    D. vaginal delivery.

    E. the use of corticosteroids.

367. *Candida albicans:*

    A. causes oral infection in neonates.

    B. is a normal commensal of the vagina.

    C. can be identified in a cervical smear.

    D. causes vulvo-vaginitis.

    E. grows on Sabouraud's medium (glucose-pentone agar).

368. The incubation period of:

    A. chickenpox is 14–21 days.

    B. rubella is 1–6 days.

    C. hepatitis B is 6 weeks to 6 months.

    D. cholera is 7–14 days.

    E. scarlet fever is 1–3 days.

369. In rubella infection:

    A. the mode of transmission is faeco-oral.

    B. the period of infectivity is from 7 days before to 7 days after the appearance of the rash.

    C. the diagnosis is usually made by viral isolation.

    D. specific IgM can take up to 21 days after exposure to appear in the blood.

    E. specific IgM persist in the blood for 6 months.

370. The period of infectivity in:

    A. chickenpox lasts until 6 days after the last crop of vesicles.

    B. rubella is confined to the rash-phase.

    C. scarlet fever is unaffected by the administration of penicillin.

    D. mumps is from 3 days before to 7 days after the appearance of the salivary swelling.

    E. diphtheria is shortened with antibiotic therapy.

371. Infection with Epstein-Barr virus can cause:

    A. shingles.

    B. infectious mononucleosis.

    C. Burkitt's lymphoma.

    D. hairy leukoplakia in immunocompromised patients.

    E. chickenpox.

372. Herpes viruses include:

    A. cytomegalovirus.

    B. Epstein-Barr virus.

    C. varicella-zoster virus.

    D. measles virus.

    E. rubella virus.

373. *Clostridium welchii:*

    A. is an anaerobe.

    B. is a normal commensal in humans.

    C. produces endospores.

    D. causes gas gangrene.

    E. is a Gram-positive bacillus.

374. **Diseases caused by spirochaetes include:**

    A. yaws.

    B. Weil's disease.

    C. Vincent's angina.

    D. trench fever.

    E. syphilis.

375. **A false positive Wassermann reaction may be caused by:**

    A. pregnancy.

    B. leprosy.

    C. glandular fever.

    D. systemic lupus erythematosus.

    E. tuberculosis.

376. **During normal pregnancy, a false positive result may be found in:**

    A. venereal disease research laboratory (VDRL) test.

    B. rapid plasma reagin (RPR) test.

    C. *Treponema pallidum* haemagglutination assay (TPHA).

    D. *Treponema pallidum* immobilization (TPI) test.

    E. Kahn test.

377. **The following infections can be transmitted to the fetus transplacentally:**

    A. toxoplasmosis.

    B. malaria.

    C. cytomegalovirus.

    D. herpes simplex.

    E. parvovirus.

378. *Neisseria gonorrhoeae:*

    A. is a normal commensal in humans.

    B. grows well in 5–10% carbon dioxide.

    C. penetrates stratified squamous epithelium.

    D. can cause infection of Skene's ducts.

    E. is found inside polymorphonuclear leucocytes in the inflammatory exudate from infected individuals.

379. *Neisseria gonorrhoeae* **can cause:**

    A. ophthalmia neonatorum.

    B. acute vulvovaginitis.

    C. pharyngitis.

    D. proctitis.

    E. urethritis.

380. **Salmonella organisms:**

    A. are lactose-fermenting organisms.

    B. cause bacillary dysentery.

    C. are Gram-positive.

    D. cause enteric fever.

    E. cause food poisoning.

381. **In the reproductive age-group the normal vaginal flora include:**

    A. *Bacteroides fragilis.*

    B. *Gardnerella vaginalis.*

    C. *Escherichia coli.*

    D. *Neisseria gonorrhoeae.*

    E. *Mycoplasma hominis.*

382. **Döderlein's bacillus is the predominant organism in the vagina of the healthy female:**

    A. at birth.

    B. during the first few days of life.

    C. in childhood.

    D. during the reproductive years.

    E. in the postmenopausal period.

383. Vaginal flora in the healthy female child can include:

A. Diphtheroids.

B. *Clostridium perfringens.*

C. *Gardnerella vaginalis.*

D. *Staphylococcus epidermidis.*

E. *Bacteroides melaninogenicus.*

384. The following are motile organisms:

A. *Shigella sonnei.*

B. *Salmonella typhi.*

C. *Clostridium welchii.*

D. *Chlamydia trachomatis.*

E. *Listeria monocytogenes.*

385. Bacteroides are:

A. anaerobes.

B. spore-forming organisms.

C. Gram-positive.

D. part of the normal flora of the mouth.

E. sensitive to metronidazole.

386. Tuberculosis of the genital tract:

A. is usually a blood-borne infection.

B. has the primary site of infection in the Fallopian tube in over 90% of cases.

C. is caused by a Gram-negative organism.

D. is treated primarily by surgery.

E. is associated with caseation.

387. The human immunodeficiency virus (HIV):

A. is a retrovirus.

B. is a DNA virus.

C. can be transmitted transplacentally.

D. contains the enzyme reverse transcriptase.

E. can be isolated using the enzyme-linked immunosorbent assay (ELISA).

388. *Actinomyces israeli:*

   A. is a normal commensal of the gut in humans.

   B. is resistant to penicillin.

   C. infection of the genital tract is associated with the presence of the intrauterine contraceptive device (IUCD).

   D. can lead to granulomatous pelvic-abdominal infection.

   E. is Gram-negative.

389. Chlamydiae:

   A. multiply by binary fission.

   B. are infectious when in the form of 'reticulate bodies'.

   C. contain ribosomes.

   D. grow in the cytoplasm of the host cell as acidophilic inclusion bodies.

   E. contain DNA and RNA.

390. Viruses:

   A. multiply by replication.

   B. contain mitochondria.

   C. are intracellular parasites.

   D. contain ribosomes.

   E. contain either DNA or RNA, but never both.

391. DNA viruses include:

   A. herpesvirus.

   B. enterovirus.

   C. poxvirus.

   D. parvovirus.

   E. rotavirus.

392. Cytomegalovirus (CMV) infection:

   A. confers life-long immunity.

   B. is usually symptomless.

   C. can be acquired transplacentally.

    D. can be acquired through blood transfusion.

    E. is due to an infection with an RNA virus.

393. **The following vaccines are contraindicated during pregnancy:**

    A. measles vaccine.

    B. poliomyelitis Sabin vaccine.

    C. diphtheria toxoids.

    D. rubella vaccine.

    E. smallpox vaccine.

394. *Trichomonas vaginalis:*

    A. infection can be transmitted by sexual intercourse.

    B. has flagellae.

    C. invades vaginal epithelium.

    D. can be detected on cervical smears.

    E. is sensitive to clotrimazole.

395. *Toxoplasma gondii:*

    A. is an intracellular protozoan.

    B. may be acquired through eating undercooked meat.

    C. infection is associated with lymphadenopathy.

    D. infection may be acquired transplacentally.

    E. is sensitive to spiramycin.

▌ MICROBIOLOGY: ANSWERS

356. AE

Bacteria replicate by simple fusion when the cell enlarges and divides into two almost equal daughter cells separated by a septum. This division is preceded by simple replication of the nucleus, which contains a ribbon of double-stranded deoxyribonucleic acid (DNA). The staining characteristics are a function of the bacterial cell wall and not the nucleus.

357. AE

Staining characteristics are one of the methods used for identifying bacteria. *Neisseria gonorrhoeae* and *Escherichia coli* are Gram-negative. *Treponema pallidum* is a spirochaete which is not stainable by Gram, but appears as a pink thread on Giemsa staining.

358. ABC

Enteric fever is caused by *Salmonella* and scarlet fever is caused by *Streptococcus pyogenes*.

359. ABE

Staphylococcus aureus is an important cause of hospital wound infections and abscesses. The majority of staphylococci isolated in hospital produce penicillinase and are thus resistant to penicillin and ampicillin; a fact which should be noted when prescribing for postoperative wound infection. These organisms are sensitive to flucloxacillin, cephalosporins, fucidin, clindamycin and gentamicin. Erysipelas is a streptococcal infection.

360. ABCDE

Beta-haemolytic streptococcus is an important cause of neonatal septicaemia, which can occur in the babies of women carrying the organism in the vagina. The baby contracts the infection either during delivery or *in utero* in cases of prolonged prelabour rupture of the amniotic membrane. The mortality of this neonatal infection is over 50%.

361. BDE

Corynebacterium diphtheriae is a Gram-positive organism. Schick's test is used to distinguish susceptible individuals from those immune to diphtheria by injecting diphtheria toxins intradermally and observing for oedema and erythema (maximum in 2–4 days) in susceptible individuals.

362. ABCD

Listeria monocytogenes is an important human pathogen, particularly during pregnancy; almost one-third of the cases occur during pregnancy (maternal, fetal) or the neonatal period. The organism is usually carried in the gut and is present in many types of food (salads, dairy products, cheese, milk, cooked chilled food, meat).

363. ACDE

Listeriosis occurs throughout pregnancy and should be considered when the mother has a pyrexial flu-like illness. Many cases, however, are asymptomatic. The fetus is usually affected, with intrauterine death occurring in up to 20% of cases.

364. ABCDE

Staphylococcus aureus can cause meningitis in predisposed patients (i.e. those with shunts).

365. BC

Condyloma lata are manifestations of secondary syphilis. Condyloma acuminata (genital warts) are caused by human papilloma virus. Lymphogranuloma venereum is caused by *Chlamydia trachomatis* and granuloma inguinale by *Calymmatobacterium granulomatis*.

366. ABCE

The incidence of vaginal thrush is markedly increased during pregnancy, particularly in the third trimester and during the summer months. After delivery, however, the incidence is greatly diminished, perhaps as a result of the cleansing effect of the lochia.

367. ABCDE

Candida albicans can be found in the vagina in up to 36% of women during pregnancy and up to 16% of non-pregnant women in the reproductive age. Neonatal oral thrush is usually due to transmission of infection from the mother's vagina, and therefore occurs more commonly in babies born to women who harbour the fungus.

368. ACE

The incubation period of rubella is 14–21 days and that of cholera is from a few hours to 5 days (average 2–3 hours).

369. BD

Rubella (or German measles, as it was first recognized as a disease separate from measles by two German physicians) is usually a mild childhood illness. In pregnancy, however, it is very important as it can lead to congenital infection and abnormalities; up to 50% of fetuses are affected if the disease is contracted in the first trimester. The virus is carried in the nasopharynx and is spread by droplets. The diagnosis is usually made by serological tests, either looking for rubella-specific IgM (which does not persist more than one month), or a rising titre of rubella antibodies.

370. ADE

In rubella the period of infectivity is from 7 days before to 7 days after the appearance of the rash. In scarlet fever it is 10 to 21 days after the onset of the rash, but can be reduced to 1 day by penicillin. It is important to advise pregnant women with contagious droplet infections not to come to the antenatal clinic (where they may infect other pregnant women) during the periods of infectivity. Other arrangements, of course, have to be made for antenatal care during those periods.

371. BCD

Chickenpox and shingles are caused by varicella-zoster virus.

372. ABC

Measles virus is a paramyxovirus and rubella virus is a togavirus.

373. ABCDE

Clostridium welchii is a common inhabitant of the intestinal tract of humans and animals. The reason why it is rarely reported as occurring in rectal swabs and stools is because these specimens are very often cultured aerobically. The rare presence of this organism in swabs from the vagina or perineum does not – on its own – imply infection, and the whole clinical picture should be considered.

374. ABCE

Syphilis is the most notable disease caused by spirochaetes
(*Treponema pallidum*). Other diseases include yaws (a granulomatous
disease involving the skin and bones and caused by *Treponema
pertenue*), Weil's disease (an infection caused by contracting *Leptospira
icterhaemohagiae* from the urine of infected rodents), and Vincent's
angina (or 'tropical ulcer' caused by *Borrelia vincenti*). Trench fever is
caused by rickettsiae and not by spirochaetes.

375. ABCDE

Wassermann reaction is a complement fixation test utilizing
cardiolipin (heart extract) antigen and is used in the diagnosis of
syphilis. Other causes of a false positive result include sleeping
sickness and malaria. The test is also positive in yaws and pinta but,
as these are infections caused by spirochaetes, they are regarded as
'true' rather than 'false' positive. A positive Wassermann reaction
necessitates confirmation by a specific test before syphilis is
confidently diagnosed.

376. ABE

Serological tests for the diagnosis of syphilis are routinely performed
in pregnancy because of the dangers of untreated syphilis to the fetus
and the potential for their complete prevention by early treatment.
Two types of test are available. The first is non-specific, can give false
positive results in pregnancy and turns negative within one year of
cure. Examples of these non-specific tests include the VDRL, RPR
and Khan tests. The second type detects antitreponemal antibodies in
the serum, is specific and tends to remain positive for life, even after
cure. Examples include TPHA, TPI and the fluorescent treponemal
antibody test (FTA-ABS). During pregnancy a test of the first type
is used for screening and, if positive, a test of the second type is
used for confirmation. Cooperation between the clinician and the
microbiologist is required for proper interpretation of the results.

377. ABCDE

Toxoplasmosis, rubella, cytomegalovirus and herpes simplex form
the acronym TORCH, and can lead to intrauterine death, growth
retardation and a variety of congenital malformations. A ' TORCH

screen' is included in the investigations of such conditions if they are otherwise unexplained.

378. BDE

Neisseria meningitidis and *Neisseria pharyngis* (but not *Neisseria gonorrhoeae*) are present in 10% of normal individuals. *Neisseria gonorrhoeae* infects columnar epithelium (e.g. endocervix) and is unable to penetrate stratified squamous epithelium (e.g. vagina); hence a cervical swab is taken to investigate suspected lower genital tract gonorrhoea.

379. ABCDE

Neisseria gonorrhoeae can cause acute vulvovaginitis in infants and young girls. This infection can spread by contact with contaminated fomites and can reach epidemic proportions in institution.

380. DE

Salmonella species are non-lactose-fermenting Gram-negative enteric rods. *S. typhi* and *S. paratyphi* cause typhoid and paratyphoid fever (enteric fever). *S. typhimurium* and *S. enteritidis* cause food poisoning. Bacillary dysentery is caused by *Shigella* species (mainly *Shigella sonnei*).

381. ABCE

In the normal postmenarchal woman there are about $10^8 - 10^9$ anaerobes/ml and about $10^7 - 10^8$ aerobes/ml of vaginal secretion. Therefore, the finding of organisms in vaginal microbiological specimens should be interpreted in conjunction with the whole clinical picture. *Neisseria gonorrhoeae* is not a normal vaginal commensal and its isolation indicates infection.

382. BD

Döderlein's bacilli are Gram-positive organisms which predominate in the normal vaginal flora during the periods of life when there is a high oestrogenic milieu. The oestrogen causes deposition of glycogen in the vaginal epithelium and Döderlein's bacillus converts the glycogen into lactic acid (which is responsible for the normal vaginal acidity; pH 4–5). At birth the vagina is sterile but within 1–2 days the oestrogen (derived from the maternal circulation *in utero*) leads to the appearance of Döderlein's bacilli.

383. ABCDE

During the years of low oestrogen before puberty the vaginal secretions are alkaline and many different organisms inhabit the vagina. At puberty, however, the oestrogenic environment is established, with the resultant deposition of glycogen in vaginal epithelium and the establishment of Döderlein's bacillus as the predominant vaginal commensal.

384. BE

Motility is one of the characteristics used in identifying different types of bacterium. *Clostridium welchii* is the only organism in the *Clostridium* genus that is non-motile. The Shigellas and the Chlamydias are all non-motile.

385. ADE

Bacteroides are Gram-negative non-sporing organisms which form part of the normal flora of the mouth, gut and vagina. They can cause bacterial vaginosis, which is a non-specific infection of the vagina characterized by a foul-smelling fishy discharge.

386. ABE

Mycobacterium tuberculosis is a Gram-positive, acid and alcohol fast, aerobic non-motile organism. Genital tuberculosis is almost always a blood-borne infection from a focus elsewhere (usually in the lungs). The treatment is primarily medical with antituberculous drugs.

387. ACD

HIV and other retroviruses are RNA viruses. Their name refers to the fact that RNA transcription proceeds in a reverse direction (RNA to DNA) before the viral genome can be incorporated into the host genome and viral replication starts. This essential retrograde step depends upon the presence of the enzyme reverse transcriptase. ELISA is used to detect HIV antibodies.

388. ACD

Actinomyces israeli is a Gram-positive mycelium-bearing anaerobic fungus which is a normal commensal of the mouth and gut. Pelvic actinomycosis was previously almost always secondary to intestinal lesions such as ruptured appendix or bowel perforation. More recently the infection is associated with IUCD, particularly those devices not containing copper. The copper in some devices seems to have a bacteriostatic effect, providing relative protection against pelvic actinomycosis. The organism is sensitive to penicillin.

389. ACE

Chlamydiae are infectious as 'elementary bodies' which are about 0.3 μm in diameter. These are phagocytosed by host cells where they develop into the larger 'reticulate bodies'. They are seen as basophilic intracellular inclusion bodies in Giemsa stained specimens.

390. ACE

Viruses are obligatory intracellular parasites which have no metabolism (or mitochondria and ribosomes) of their own and cannot reproduce independently of the host cell.

391. ACD

Unlike other micro-organisms, viruses contain either DNA or RNA, but never both. Enterovirus, rotavirus, reovirus, myxovirus and arbovirus are examples of RNA viruses. Adenovirus and papovavirus are examples of DNA viruses.

392. BCD

CMV is a herpesvirus (DNA virus). After a primary infection it has the ability of latency with subsequent reactivation to produce a recurrent infection. After a primary infection during pregnancy there is about a 40% chance of transmitting the infection to the fetus. CMV is thought to be the commonest intrauterine infection in Great Britain; 0.4%–2.2% of newborn babies have congenital CMV infection and one in five of these babies will be damaged. The risk in recurrent infection is thought to be less than that, but it is still possible.

393. ABDE

Live viral or bacterial vaccines are contraindicated during pregnancy for fear of fetal infection. These include rubella, measles, smallpox, yellow fever and live oral (Sabin) poliomyelitis. Toxoids (e.g. tetanus, diphtheria) and the inactivated Salk poliomyelitis vaccine can be safely used during pregnancy.

394. ABD

Vaginal infection with *Trichomonas vaginalis* is common, with about two million cases treated annually in Britain. The organism (a protozoan) does not invade the epithelium and is sensitive to metronidazole.

395. ABCDE

Congenital toxoplasmosis complicates about 0.5% of all pregnancies in Britain. The infection is usually acquired by the mother through eating undercooked meat or contact with cat litter. The rate of congenital infection is related to the trimester during which the mother is infected; the lowest incidence (25%) is in the first trimester, and the highest (65%) is in the third trimester.

12

Pathology and Immunology

396. Collagen:

  A. has a trihelical structure.

  B. type III is the main type found in fetal tissue.

  C. type II is found in early scar tissue in the adult.

  D. is a polysaccharide.

  E. is secreted by fibroblasts.

397. Paget's disease of the bone is:

  A. localized to the tibia in most cases.

  B. more common in women than men.

  C. associated with the development of osteogenic sarcoma.

  D. a recognized cause of high output cardiac failure.

  E. associated with raised levels of plasma alkaline phosphatase.

398. Sarcoidosis is associated with:

  A. caseation.

  B. giant cell infiltration.

  C. uveitis.

  D. hypocalcaemia.

  E. hypergammaglobulinaemia.

399. Hyperpigmentation of the skin occurs in:

- A. pregnancy.
- B. Addison's disease.
- C. tyrosinase deficiency.
- D. melanosis coli.
- E. haemochromatosis.

400. Squamous metaplasia can occur in:

- A. the gall bladder.
- B. the pelvis of the kidney.
- C. bronchi.
- D. the cervix.
- E. the urinary bladder.

401. The intestine in Crohn's disease is characterized by:

- A. regional lymphadenopathy.
- B. thin walls.
- C. narrow lumen.
- D. mucosal ulceration.
- E. noncaseating granulomatous lesions.

402. Fluid pus:

- A. is acidic.
- B. clots on standing.
- C. contains dead polymorphs.
- D. contains fibrin.
- E. does not usually contain live micro-organisms.

403. Granulomatous lesions are found in:

- A. rhinoscleroma.
- B. bilharziasis.
- C. leprosy.
- D. syphilis.
- E. gonorrhoea.

404. Features of the secondary stage of syphilis include:

A. mucous patches.

B. vesicular skin rash.

C. condyloma lata.

D. aortitis.

E. epitrochlear lymphadenopathy.

405. Characteristically, the placenta of a baby with congenital syphilis:

A. is infiltrated with plasma cells.

B. is small in size.

C. is infiltrated with lymphocytes.

D. contains a chancre.

E. has endarteritis obliterans.

406. The syphilitic chancre:

A. can appear on the cervix.

B. is painless.

C. is associated with painful regional lymphadenopathy.

D. is infectious.

E. appears only on genital organs.

407. Tissues which are particularly sensitive to the effects of ionizing radiation include:

A. germinal epithelium in the gonads.

B. bones.

C. muscles.

D. gastro-intestinal epithelium.

E. central nervous system.

408. Long-term effects of ionizing radiation include:

A. osteosarcoma.

B. chronic myeloid leukaemia.

C. squamous cell carcinoma of the skin.

D. ovarian failure.

E. aspermia.

409. The local response to acute inflammation includes:

 A. vasoconstriction.

 B. slowing of the circulation.

 C. vasodilatation.

 D. increased capillary permeability.

 E. decreased osmotic pressure of the interstitial fluid.

410. The acute inflammatory exudate:

 A. contains more than 3% protein.

 B. does not clot.

 C. contains immunoglobulins.

 D. contains polymorphonuclear leucocytes.

 E. has specific gravity of less than 1010.

411. The 'cardinal' signs of inflammation include:

 A. pallor.

 B. pain.

 C. atrophy.

 D. loss of function.

 E. lymphadenopathy.

412. Characteristically there is monocytosis in:

 A. influenza.

 B. parasitic infection.

 C. malaria.

 D. typhoid fever.

 E. suppurative inflammation.

413. The polymorphonuclear leucocytes:

 A. are highly motile.

 B. contain lysozymes.

 C. have a half-life of 3 days.

 D. contain receptors for F_c protein.

 E. are the precursors of pus cells.

414. Causes of neonatal jaundice include:

    A. ampicillin therapy.

    B. congenital toxoplasmosis.

    C. ABO haemolytic diseases of the newborn.

    D. spherocytosis.

    E. rhesus iso-immunization.

415. Tumours arising from the germinal epithelium of the ovary include:

    A. Brenner's tumour.

    B. serous cystadenoma.

    C. arrhenoblastoma.

    D. dysgerminoma.

    E. papillary cystadenocarcinoma.

416. The following tumours of the ovary are hormone-secreting:

    A. theca cell tumours.

    B. solid teratoma.

    C. dysgerminoma.

    D. arrhenoblastoma.

    E. dermoid cyst.

417. *Pseudomyxoma peritonei* **is associated with:**

    A. large bowel carcinoma.

    B. mucocele of the appendix.

    C. mucinous tumours of the ovary.

    D. good response to radiotherapy.

    E. solid ovarian tumours.

418. An embolus can be formed of:

    A. air.

    B. parasitic organisms.

    C. amniotic fluid particles.

    D. fat.

    E. tumour cells.

419. Fatty change:

    A. can occur in the liver.

    B. can occur in the kidney.

    C. leads to atrophy of the affected organ.

    D. can result from chloroform poisoning.

    E. can result from excess choline.

420. Liver cirrhosis:

    A. is characterized by preservation of lobular hepatic architecture.

    B. can be a consequence of carcinoma of the head of the pancreas.

    C. can result from portal hypertension.

    D. is a cause of gynaecomastia.

    E. is associated with increased incidence of hepatoma.

421. Causes of haemoptysis include:

    A. benign tumours of the lung.

    B. portal hypertension.

    C. pulmonary tuberculosis.

    D. acute gastritis.

    E. mitral stenosis.

422. Benign tumours include:

    A. myxoma.

    B. rhabdomyoma.

    C. haemangioendothelioma.

    D. myoblastoma.

    E. basal cell epithelioma.

423. Eosinophilia is caused by:

    A. tuberculosis.

    B. polyarteritis nodosa.

    C. bronchial asthma.

    D. malaria.

    E. measles.

424. **Polycythaemia is associated with:**

    A. benzene poisoning.

    B. cyanotic congenital heart disease.

    C. hypernephroma.

    D. cerebellar angioma.

    E. acute malaria.

425. **Phaeochromocytoma:**

    A. is usually a malignant tumour.

    B. can only be found in the adrenal medulla.

    C. secretes catecholamines.

    D. is usually encapsulated.

    E. is associated with severe hypertension.

426. **Amyloidosis:**

    A. occurs in the tongue.

    B. is associated with multiple myeloma.

    C. stains with Congo red dye.

    D. can lead to bowel ulceration.

    E. is a type of coagulative necrosis.

427. **Wound healing can be impaired by:**

    A. gapping of the edges.

    B. infection.

    C. vitamin C deficiency.

    D. testosterone.

    E. ultraviolet light.

428. **Carcinoma of the prostate:**

    A. is usually an adenocarcinoma.

    B. leads to osteolytic bone metastases.

    C. is responsive to hormonal treatment.

    D. is associated with raised alkaline phosphatase.

    E. is a complication of benign nodular hyperplasia of the prostate.

429. Breast carcinoma:

    A. can occur in males.

    B. is more common in nulliparous than in parous women.

    C. is rare before the age of 30.

    D. is more common in women who breast-fed than in those who did not.

    E. usually originates in the upper outer quadrant of the breast.

430. Major histocompatibility complex (MHC) antigens:

    A. are genetically coded on chromosome 8.

    B. are abundant in normal trophoblastic tissue.

    C. subtype HLA,DR is present on the plasma membrane of macrophages.

    D. are unique for each individual.

    E. are glycoproteins.

431. Immunoglobulins IgG:

    A. cross the placenta.

    B. of fetal origin are secreted from 28 weeks gestation.

    C. are produced in the primary immune response.

    D. have some antiviral activity.

    E. are produced by plasma cells.

432. Immunoglobulin IgA is present in:

    A. bronchial secretions.

    B. colostrum.

    C. lacrimal fluid.

    D. saliva.

    E. intestinal secretions.

433. Haemolytic disease of the newborn (HDN) could be due to:

    A. anti-D antibodies.

    B. anti-Kell antibodies.

    C. anti-Lewis antibodies.

    D. anti-A antibodies.

    E. anti-B antibodies.

434. **During normal pregnancy there is:**

    A. exaggerated cell-mediated immunity.

    B. an increase in the number of helper T lymphocytes.

    C. an inversion of the normal T to B lymphocytes ratio in the first trimester.

    D. neutrophilia.

    E. an increase in IgD.

435. **Human milk contains:**

    A. Immunoglobulins.

    B. T lymphocytes.

    C. B lymphocytes.

    D. lactoferrin.

    E. anti-staphylococcal factor.

436. **In the fetus:**

    A. IgM can be of maternal origin.

    B. T lymphocytes start to develop at about 8 weeks of intrauterine life.

    C. the liver and spleen produce B lymphocytes.

    D. at term IgG blood levels may be higher than in the mother.

    E. IgG is the first type of immunoglobulins to be produced in large quantities.

437. **Examples of type I hypersensitivity reactions include:**

    A. Koch's phenomenon.

    B. allergic contact dermatitis.

    C. hay fever.

    D. anaphylactic shock.

    E. allergic rhinitis.

438. In complete hydatidiform mole:
- **A.** the karyotype is usually 46,XX.
- **B.** an X chromosome is often of maternal origin.
- **C.** villi are characteristically vascular.
- **D.** there are cytotrophoblastic and syncytial elements.
- **E.** vagina bleeding is the most common presenting symptom.

439. T lymphocytes:
- **A.** are formed in the thymus gland.
- **B.** form about 75% of circulating lymphocytes.
- **C.** have high nuclear-cytoplasmic ratio.
- **D.** mediate cellular immunity.
- **E.** secrete lymphokines.

440. The following mediators are stored within granules in mast cells:
- **A.** histamine.
- **B.** heparin.
- **C.** thromboxane.
- **D.** tryptase.
- **E.** leukotrienes C_4.

▌ PATHOLOGY AND IMMUNOLOGY: ANSWERS

396. ABE

Collagen is a protein providing structural integrity to tissues. It has four biochemical types. Type I is found in bone, tendon and dermis. It is the main type found in adults and forms more than 50% of total body protein. Type II is found in cartilage. Type III is the fetal collagen and is replaced after birth by type I. In the adult, type III is present in small amounts in cardiovascular tissue and synovium and also appears in early scar tissue (as reticulin). Type IV is the basement membrane collagen.

397. CDE

Paget's disease of the bone (osteitis deformans) is characterized by softening, enlargement, and bowing of bones. In most cases it is generalized, affecting the skull, vertebrae and bones of the leg. Rarely it is localized to the tibia. It is more common in men and develops after the age of 40. There is increased vascularity in the affected areas and, rarely, widespread arteriovenous shunts leading to high-output cardiac failure.

398. BCE

Sarcoidosis is a rare generalized chronic granulomatous disease of unknown cause. The mediastinal and superficial lymph nodes, lungs, liver, spleen, skin, eyes, parotid glands and phalangeal bones are most frequently affected and infiltrated with epitheloid and giant cells (similar to tuberculous follicles) but without caseation. Calcium metabolism may be disturbed causing hypercalcaemia.

399. ABE

Tyrosinase catalyses the oxidation of tyrosine to dihydroxyphenylalanine, which is a precursor of melanin. Tyrosinase deficiency, therefore, leads to hypopigmentation. In melanosis coli there is hyperpigmentation of the mucous membranes of the large intestines and the appendix, but no skin hyperpigmentation.

400. ABCDE

In squamous metaplasia the native epithelium is transformed into a more resistant type of epithelium (stratified squamous) as a result of chronic irritation (mechanical or inflammatory).

401. ACDE

In Crohn's disease (regional ileitis) the intestinal wall is thickened with 'cobble stone' appearance of the mucous membrane, which is raised by the underlying inflammation and oedema. Short lengths of the intestine are affected, leaving normal bowel between, i.e. skip lesions.

402. CD

Fluid pus is thick alkaline fluid which does not clot. It is formed of pus cells (dead polymorphs), liquefied necrotic tissue and debris, oedema fluid, fibrin and the causative organisms, many of them still alive.

403. ABCD

Granulomas are a type of chronic inflammation in which the specific inflammatory cells form tumour-like masses. They also include tuberculosis, actinomycosis and sarcoidosis.

404. ACE

Features of secondary syphilis include: syphilitic skin rash (which appears as macules, papules and pustules but no vesicles); leucoderma; alopecia; mucous patches; condyloma lata; generalized lymphadenopathy, characteristically in the epitrochlear and posterior cervical groups; and bony lesions. Aortitis is a feature of tertiary syphilis.

405. ACE

The placenta in congenital syphilis is enlarged, firm and pale in colour. The chorionic villi are swollen and infiltrated by plasma cells and lymphocytes with endarteritis obliterans of their vessels. Although congenital syphilis can be regarded as a combination of the features of secondary and tertiary acquired syphilis in the baby with the primary lesion in the placenta, there is no characteristic placental chancre.

406. ABD

The chancre is a very firm painless nodule which ulcerates and becomes very infectious. The regional lymph nodes are enlarged, indurated and also painless. The commonest sites for the chancre are the genital organs, but it can also appear on extragenital sites, such as the lips, tongue and nipple.

407. AD

The higher the normal mitotic rate of the exposed cells, the greater their sensitivity to ionizing radiation. Haemopoietic, germinal and gastro-intestinal epithelium are particularly sensitive. Bones, muscles and central nervous system tissue are relatively radioresistant.

408. ABCD

Ionizing radiation treatment can have long-term carcinogenic effects on exposed tissues. Ovarian tissue can be irreversibly damaged with doses of 600–1000 cGy. Testicular tissue can be similarly damaged, leading to azoospermia (no spermatozoa in the ejaculate). Aspermia (no ejaculate) does not usually result. Men who will undergo testicular irradiation should be counselled regarding sperm freezing and banking prior to their radiotherapy.

409. ABCD

In acute inflammation there is a transient vasoconstriction initially, which is rapidly followed by arteriolar vasodilatation. Slowing of the circulation then follows and may even amount to complete stasis. The increased capillary permeability and osmotic pressure of the interstitial fluid contribute to the escape of the plasma to the interstitial space and the formation of the inflammatory exudate.

410. ACD

The inflammatory exudate contains fibrin and, therefore, clots on standing. It has a high cellular and protein content and a specific gravity of more than 1015.

411. BD

The 'cardinal' signs of inflammation appear mainly in acute inflammation and are: redness (rubor), hotness (calor), swelling (tumour), pain (dolor) and loss of function.

412. ABC

In parasitic infections there is usually eosinophilia, while in suppurative inflammation there is neutrophilia. In malaria, typhoid fever and influenza there is monocytosis with overall leucopenia.

413. ABDE

Polymorphonuclear leucocytes are the main inflammatory cells of acute inflammation. They are short-lived, with a half-life of about 7 hours. They have a multilobed nucleus and a cytoplasm with neutrophilic granules (lysozymes and lactoferrin) and azurophil granules (containing bactericidal enzymes). Dead polymorphs are pus cells.

414. BCDE

Although *in vitro* studies have shown that many drugs (including ampicillin) interfere with bilirubin-albumin binding, this effect has been shown to be important *in vivo* only in the case of sulphonamides.

415. ABE

Epithelial ovarian tumours account for more than 90% of cases of ovarian malignancy. Arrhenoblastoma arises from the ovarian stroma and dysgerminoma arises from the germ cells.

416. ACD

Functioning tumours of the ovary include granulosa cell tumours, theca cell tumours, arrhenoblastoma, dysgerminoma and Brenner's tumour.

417. ABC

Pseudomyxoma peritonei is a rare complication of spontaneous perforation of mucinous tumours in the peritoneal cavity. There is widespread peritoneal seeding of mucinous epithelium and a massive accumulation of thick mucinous material. It is a debilitating condition, with many patients dying from cachexia and no good response to radiotherapy or chemotherapy. The most satisfactory treatment is multiple surgical procedures to relieve symptoms.

418. ABCDE

An embolus can be formed of a detached part of thrombus, tumour cells, bilharzia ova, *Entamoeba histolytica*, air, fat, trophoblastic cells, amniotic fluid particles and atheromatous lesions.

419. ABD

Fatty change is a disturbance in fat metabolism in which the fat that is usually used for metabolic purposes is inadequately utilized, remains free in the cytoplasm and accumulates as large droplets of fat. It can occur in liver, kidney and heart, which become enlarged, soft and yellow in colour. Causes include bacterial toxins, tissue anoxia, exogenous toxins (carbon tetrachloride, chloroform) and deficiency of lipotropic factors such as choline.

420. BDE

Liver cirrhosis is characterized by liver injury with necrosis and degeneration followed by regeneration of the liver cells and increased amount of fibrosis, resulting in loss of the lobular hepatic architecture. Cirrhosis can lead to portal hypertension.

421. ACE

Haemoptysis is coughing of blood and haematemesis is vomiting of blood. Portal hypertension (leading to oesophageal varices) and acute gastritis can lead to haematemesis.

422. ABD

Haemangioendothelioma is a rare malignant tumour of blood vessels occurring more commonly in the skin and liver of young people and appears as a rounded firm greyish pink nodule. Basal cell epithelioma (rodent ulcer) is a locally malignant tumour arising from the basal cells of the skin of areas exposed to the sunshine, particularly the face and neck.

423. BC

Tuberculosis, malaria (and other protozoal infections such as leishmaniasis and trypanosomiasis) and measles (and other viral infections such as influenza, smallpox and viral hepatitis) cause leucopenia.

424. BCD

Benzene poisoning can lead to anaplastic anaemia and acute malaria can lead to haemolytic anaemia.

425. CDE

Phaeochromocytoma is a rare tumour which is usually benign and arises from the chromaffin cells in the adrenal medulla or the retroperitoneal tissue. It is a recognized cause of severe hypertension in pregnancy and has a high mortality rate. Measurement of urinary vanillylmandelic acid (VMA) is used to screen for this condition in suspected cases.

426. ABCD

Amyloidosis is the condition in which there is deposition of 'amyloid material' (complex mucopolysaccharide containing globulins) in the connective tissue stroma and the walls of blood vessels of certain tissues and organs. It is a rare complication of chronic infection, collagen disease and multiple myeloma.

427. ABC

Testosterone and other anabolic steroids increase the speed of wound healing, as does the exposure to ultraviolet light.

428. AC

Carcinoma of the prostate usually occurs over the age of 60 and is often associated with benign nodular hyperplasia although there is no direct relation between the two diseases. It characteristically leads to osteosclerotic bone metastasis and is associated with raised levels of acid phosphatase.

429. ACE

One per cent of cases of breast carcinoma occur in males. In females, it is rare before the age of 30, with a peak between 40 and 50 years. It is more common in parous than in nulliparous women and in those who did not breast-feed.

430. CDE

MHC are genetically coded on chromosome 6. They are absent from the normal trophoblastic tissues which may partially explain why the fetus (which is a sort of an allogenic transplant in the mother) is not normally rejected.

431. ADE

IgG is the only class of immunoglobulins that crosses the placenta (by an active process). Babies do not start producing their own IgG until the maternal IgG (which has been transfused transplacentally *in utero*) has been catabolized at about 3–4 months of age. IgM is the immunoglobulin of primary immune response.

432. ABCDE

IgA is the immunoglobulin that predominates in the internal and external secretions of the body and provides antibody activity at sites that are not readily accessible to other immunoglobulins.

433. ABDE

In the past rhesus anti-D antibodies used to be the commonest cause of HDN, but since the development and widespread use of anti-D immunoglobulins the incidence has become far less; currently ABO HDN is 2–4 times commoner than rhesus HDN. Anti-Lewis antibodies are not haemolytic as the antigen is adsorbed from the plasma and is not an intrinsic part of the red blood cell membrane.

434. CDE

During pregnancy the cell-mediated immunity is slightly depressed and the number of helper T cells is reduced. These changes, coupled with the fact that the trophoblasts do not exhibit MHC antigens, may partially explain the lack of rejection of the fetal 'transplant' in the mother in normal pregnancy.

435. ABCDE

Breast-feeding is a route of transferring passive immunity from the mother to the baby. Milk IgA and lymphocytes usually show activities directed towards gut pathogens and lactoferrin sequesters the iron needed by those pathogens.

436. BCD

The only class of immunoglobulins to cross the placenta is IgG. Any IgM in the fetus must be of fetal origin. Maternal IgG is transferred to the fetus by an active process and exerts a negative feedback on the fetal ability to produce its own native IgG. This negative feedback effect starts to disappear at 3–4 months of age, the time needed for maternal IgG to be catabolized.

437. CDE

In type I hypersensitivity reaction there is IgE production instead of IgG in response to certain allergens. This is due to a genetic defect in the individual concerned. IgE-antigen complex leads to mast cell membrane destabilization and release of vasoactive mediators such as histamine. Koch's phenomenon and allergic contact dermatitis are examples of type IV cell-mediated hypersensitivity reactions.

438. ADE

In the classic complete mole the 46,XX genome is formed by the fertilization of an empty egg by a normal spermatozoon carrying a 23X set of chromosomes, and this set of paternal chromosomes duplicates to form the homozygous diploid genome. The villi are characteristically avascular.

439. BCDE

T lymphocytes are derived from precursor stem cells in the bone marrow, which have matured under the influence of a hormone or factor produced by the epithelial cells of the thymus gland.

440. ABD

Although thromboxane and leukotrienes C_4 are not stored in the mast cells, they are newly synthesized as a result of mast cell degranulation such as in anaphylactic shock.

13

Statistics and Biophysics

▌ STATISTICS AND BIOPHYSICS: QUESTIONS

441. A double-blind clinical trial can be used to compare:

   A. labetalol and methyldopa in the treatment of pre-eclampsia.

   B. hysterectomy and endometrial resection in the treatment of menorrhagia.

   C. out-patient and in-patient management of asymptomatic placenta praevia.

   D. cervical cerclage and no treatment in suspected cervical incompetence.

   E. aspirin and placebo in the prevention of pre-eclampsia.

442. In a sample of 400 female university students, the mean weight was 63 kg and the standard deviation was 2.4. If the weights had normal distribution:

   A. the expected modal height would be 63.

   B. the degree of freedom was 200.

   C. the standard error of the mean would be 0.12.

   D. the variance would be 4.8.

   E. 66% of the students in the sample would be expected to weigh between 60.6 and 65.4 kg.

443. In a sample of 100 pre-eclamptic pregnant women, if the mean serum albumin is 24 g/L, the standard deviation is 4 and the distribution is normal:

   A. the variance is 16.

   B. 95% of the values will fall between 16 and 32.

   C. the standard error of the mean is 0.4.

   D. it is unlikely that any value will be 33.

   E. the measured variable (serum albumin) is a ratio variable.

444. In any set of observations:

   A. the mean is always less than the mode.

   B. half of the observations are greater than the median.

   C. if the data are skewed to the right, the median is less than the mean.

   D. the mode is always the most frequently occurring value.

   E. the variance is the square root of the standard deviation.

445. In a set of observations with skewness to the right, the median is:

   A. less than the mode.

   B. the value that half of the data points fall above it and half below it.

   C. a better representative of the data than the mean is.

   D. the best measure of central tendency in ordinal data.

   E. always represented by one of the data points.

446. Examples of nominal data include:

   A. ethnic origin data.

   B. gender data.

   C. cancer staging data.

   D. serum uric acid data.

   E. height data.

447. In statistical significance tests:

A. a P value < 0.01 is more significant than a P value < 0.05.

B. if the difference between the response to two drugs yielded a P value 0.001, then there is a clinically significant difference between them.

C. a P value > 0.05 is usually taken to indicate that the difference in the results is unlikely to be due to chance.

D. non-parametric tests can be used in normally distributed data.

E. if a difference is significant with a P value < 0.05 then the null hypothesis is false.

448. An antenatal screening test for pre-eclampsia was evaluated in 100 primigravid women, and 20 of them were screen-positive. At the end of the study ten women in total developed pre-eclampsia; only five of them were out of the 20 screen-positive women. The:

A. sensitivity of the test is 50%.

B. specificity of the test is 10%.

C. positive predictive value of the test is 25%.

D. negative predictive value of the test is 5%.

E. test would be expected to have similar performance if applied to the whole pregnant population (primigravid and multigravid).

449. The perinatal mortality rate:

A. represents the stillbirth rate and the total neonatal death rate.

B. in England includes babies born dead after 24 weeks gestation.

C. uses the number of live births as a denominator.

D. is reduced by antenatal detection and termination of fetuses with lethal congenital anomalies.

E. only includes babies delivered after 24 weeks gestation.

450. In a set of data with normal (Gaussian) distribution:

    A. the mean is equal to the median.

    B. 99% of values would be expected to lie within the mean $\pm 2.58 \times$ standard deviation.

    C. the coefficient of variation expresses the standard deviation as a percentage of the mean.

    D. the skewness is usually $\geq +5$.

    E. parametric significance tests can be used.

451. In diagnostic ultrasound:

    A. the range of frequencies used is $1-10\,\text{kHz}$.

    B. depth of penetration increases with increased frequency.

    C. resolution increases with increased frequency.

    D. attenuation increases with increased frequency.

    E. wave velocity increases with increased frequency.

452. In ionizing radiations:

    A. a proton has a negative charge.

    B. an alpha particle has two positive charges.

    C. beta particles are electrons.

    D. a positron has two positive charges.

    E. the energy of a gamma quantum is proportional to its frequency.

▍ STATISTICS AND BIOPHYSICS: ANSWERS

441. AE

In a double-blind trial, to avoid bias and placebo effect, neither the patient nor the physician knows what treatment is being administered. This is possible when comparing two drugs or comparing a drug with a placebo as was the case in the CLASP (collaborative low dose aspirin study in pregnancy) trial.

442. ACE

As the sample was normally distributed, the mean would be expected to be equal to the mode. The degree of freedom is the number in the sample minus 1 (400 − 1 = 399). The standard deviation (2.4) is the square root of the variance (5.76). Of the sample, 66% would be expected to fall within the mean ± standard deviation. The standard error of the mean = standard deviation/square root of the sample size = 2.4/20.

443. AC

In any normally distributed data, 95% of the sample would be expected to fall within the mean ± 2 × standard deviation. For the example in the question this is 16 to 32. However, item 'B' is false because it says that the '... values *will* fall...'. Statistical methods can tell us what is expected to happen, but not necessarily what will happen. If item 'B' was '...value *would be expected* to fall...' then it would have been true. It is very important to understand this fine but vital difference when interpreting statistical results.

444. BCD

If the data were skewed to the left then the mean (average) would be less than the mode (the most frequently occurring value). The standard deviation is the square root of the variance.

445. BCD

With a skew to the right the median is greater than the mode but less than the mean. It is the measure of central tendency least affected by skewness and, therefore, more useful than the mean in such cases. If there is an odd number of values, then the middle one (i.e. half of the data points fall above it and half below it) is the median. If there is an even number of values, then the average of the two middle ones is the median and in such case the median is not represented by one of the data points.

446. AB

Nominal data consist of named categories (e.g. male/female, Caucasian/Asian/African) with no implied order among the categories. When the different categories can be ranked in order (e.g. stages of cancer) the data are called ordered data. In ordered data the difference between the categories cannot be considered equal, i.e. stage II endometrial cancer is worse than, but not necessarily twice as bad as, stage I. If the difference between the different values is equal (e.g. physical and biochemical measurements) the data are called ratio data.

447. AD

Significance tests tell us if the difference is likely (null hypothesis accepted) or unlikely (null hypothesis rejected) to be due to chance. Rejecting the null hypothesis on the balance of probability is not the same as finding it false, which cannot be done by statistics. The conventional P value < 0.05 means that there is a less than 1 in 20 chance for the difference to have arisen by chance. It is very important to understand that statistical significance does not necessarily mean clinical significance.

448. AC

Table 1 and the following definitions illustrate the meaning of these commonly used terms.

Sensitivity ($=a/a+c$) is the probability that the test will be positive if the condition is present. *Specificity* ($=d/b+d$) is the probability that the test will be negative if the condition is absent. *Positive predictive value* ($=a/a+b$) is the probability that the condition is present if the test is positive. *Negative predictive value* ($=d/c+d$) is the probability that the condition is absent if the test is negative. The test will not have the same performance in the whole population because the incidence of the condition (pre-eclampsia) is different between

Table 1 A typical 2×2 table used in descriptive statistical calculations

	Women having the condition	Women not having the condition
screen-positive	true positive (a)	false positive (b)
screen-negative	false negative (c)	true negative (d)

the study population (primigravid) and the whole population (primigravid and multigravid).

449. BD

The perinatal mortality rate (PMR) includes stillbirths (babies born with no signs of life after 24 weeks gestation) and early neonatal deaths (babies born with signs of life at any gestational age and dying within the first week of life). The stillbirth definition has changed in England in late 1992 to reflect the increased survival at lower gestational ages; the previous limit of 28 weeks is now set at 24 weeks. The denominator for the PMR is the total births (live and stillborn). The term 'crude' PMR is sometimes used to describe the total PMR, and the 'corrected' PMR to describe the rate after excluding those babies who died as a result of lethal congenital abnormalities.

450. ABCE

The skewness refers to how much and in what direction the data deviate from the normal Gaussian distribution. Normal distribution has skewness equal to or nearing 0. A distribution skewed to the right has positive skewness, and that skewed to the left has negative skewness.

451. CD

Diagnostic ultrasound uses frequencies in the range 1–10 MHz. Using higher frequencies (e.g. 7.5 MHz) leads to better resolution. However, the higher the frequency the less the depth of penetration; vaginal transducers (which can get closer to the observed structure) can use higher frequencies than abdominal transducers. Higher frequencies also lead to more attenuation of the ultrasound waves, such that the upper working limit of diagnostic ultrasound is 10 MHz. Ultrasound velocity in any given medium is constant.

452. BCE

A proton has one positive charge and a mass equal to about 2000 electrons. A positron has one positive charge and a mass of one electron.

14

Practice Exams

The following 180 questions are similar to the Part 1 questions in both style and content. They are arranged in three 60-question papers. The answers are provided at the end of this chapter, but before looking them up you are advised to try to answer the questions from your knowledge. Try to practise against the clock, giving 2 hours for each paper.

▌ Paper 1 (Questions 1–60):

1. The ureter in the adult female:
   - A. crosses under the uterine artery.
   - B. is ectodermal in origin.
   - C. crosses under the genito-femoral nerve.
   - D. crosses under the ovarian vessels.
   - E. has a retroperitoneal course.

2. The following arteries are derived from the anterior division of the internal iliac artery:
   - A. uterine.
   - B. ovarian.
   - C. lateral sacral.
   - D. internal pudendal.
   - E. inferior gluteal.

3. The femoral ring:
   - A. is the abdominal end of the femoral canal.
   - B. has the lacunar ligament as a boundary.

  C. has the femoral artery as a boundary.

  D. has the inguinal ligament as a boundary.

  E. is relatively larger in the male than the female.

4. **The lesser sciatic foramen:**

  A. transmits the inferior gluteal nerve.

  B. has the sacrospinous ligament as a boundary.

  C. transmits the inferior pudendal nerve.

  D. has the sacrotuberous ligament as a boundary.

  E. transmits the tendon of obturator internus muscle.

5. **The long saphenous vein:**

  A. lies below the deep fascia.

  B. originates in the lateral end of the dorsal venous arch of the foot.

  C. passes in front of the lateral malleolus.

  D. is joined by the superficial circumflex iliac vein.

  E. is accompanied in the thigh by the saphenous nerve.

6. **The following open into the prostatic urethra:**

  A. the vas deferens.

  B. the ducts of the bulbo-urethral glands.

  C. the ducts of the seminal vesicles.

  D. the ejaculatory ducts.

  E. the prostatic ductules.

7. **The superficial inguinal ring:**

  A. transmits the ilio-inguinal nerve.

  B. is an opening in the external oblique aponeurosis.

  C. may transmit an indirect inguinal hernia.

  D. is circular in shape.

  E. may transmit a direct inguinal hernia.

8. **The pudendal canal:**

  A. is formed by the obturator fascia.

  B. is a continuation of the obturator canal.

    C. transmits the obturator artery.

    D. is situated in the lateral wall of the ischio-rectal fossa.

    E. terminates by opening into the superficial perineal pouch.

9. **The following arteries are direct branches of the superior mesenteric artery:**

    A. the right colic artery.

    B. the ileo-colic.

    C. the hepatic artery.

    D. the splenic artery.

    E. the middle colic artery.

10. **In the femoral triangle:**

    A. the femoral vein separates the femoral artery from the adductor longus muscle.

    B. the lateral border is formed by the medial margin of the sartorius muscle.

    C. part of the floor is formed by the psoas and pectineus muscles.

    D. the medial border is formed by the lateral margin of the adductor longus muscle.

    E. the femoral nerve is medial to the femoral artery.

11. **Sites of anastomoses between the systemic and portal circulations include:**

    A. the anterior abdominal wall.

    B. the bare area of the liver.

    C. the duodeno-jejunal flexure.

    D. the lower end of the oesophagus.

    E. the wall of the anal canal.

12. **A femoral hernia:**

    A. has the ilio-tibial tract as a covering.

    B. may pass through the obturator canal.

    C. has the femoral septum as a covering.

D. may ascend in the superficial fascia in front of the inguinal ligament.

E. has the stretched lacunar ligament as a covering.

13. The rectum:

A. ends beyond the tip of the coccyx.

B. has a venous drainage to the systemic circulation.

C. is suspended by a mesentery in its upper two-thirds.

D. begins at the level of the first sacral vertebra.

E. is supplied by the pelvic splanchnic nerves.

14. The amnion:

A. is surrounded by the chorion.

B. is derived from the blastocyst.

C. in a monozygotic twin pregnancy may be separated from its fellow by the chorion.

D. covers the fetal surface of the placenta.

E. separates from the decidua in the third stage of labour.

15. In the development of the female genital tract:

A. the Fallopian tube is derived from the mesonephric duct.

B. the clitoris is derived from the genital tubercle.

C. the ovarian ligament is derived from the gubernaculum.

D. the labium minor is derived from the urogenital fold.

E. the uterus is derived from the metanephric duct.

16. The following structures are of ectodermal origin:

A. lens of the eye.

B. anterior lobe of the pituitary gland.

C. mammary duct tissue.

D. adrenal cortex.

E. amniotic membrane.

17. The following are situated between the layers of the lesser omentum:

A. left gastric artery.

B. splenic artery.

   C. bile duct.

   D. portal vein.

   E. right gastro-epiploic artery.

18. **The diaphragm:**

   A. is supplied by the phrenic nerve on its inferior surface.

   B. has its caval opening opposite the 8th thoracic vertebra.

   C. has its aortic opening opposite the 10th thoracic vertebra.

   D. contracts during forced expiration.

   E. has the aorta, the azygos vein and the thoracic duct passing through its aortic opening.

19. **Serum albumin levels were measured in 100 patients with severe pre-eclampsia. The data had a normal (Gaussian) distribution, the mean was 24 g/l and the standard deviation was 4. The following statements are correct:**

   A. the variance is 16.

   B. 95% of the values will be between 16 and 32.

   C. the standard error is 0.4.

   D. the true mean is expected to be between 23.2 and 24.8.

   E. it is unlikely that any of the serum albumin values will be 33.

20. **In the statistical analysis of any group of numerical observations:**

   A. the mean is always less than the mode.

   B. half of the observations are greater than the median.

   C. if the data are skewed to the right, the mean is less than the median.

   D. the mode is the most frequently occurring value.

   E. the variance is equal to the square root of the standard deviation.

21. **The action of cortisol includes:**

   A. increased lipolysis.

   B. insulin antagonism.

   C. reduced gluconeogenesis.

    D. immunosuppression.

    E. increased sodium excretion.

22. Androgens are produced or secreted in the normal female by:

    A. the ovaries.

    B. the hypothalamus.

    C. the adrenal gland.

    D. adipose tissue.

    E. the pituitary gland.

23. Thyrotrophin (TSH):

    A. increases both the synthesis and secretion of thyroid hormones.

    B. is secreted from the acidophil cells of the anterior pituitary.

    C. its secretion is increased by somatostatin.

    D. binds to a cell membrane receptor in the thyroid gland.

    E. has increased secretion in primary myxoedema.

24. The following hormones in the fetal circulation are predominantly of maternal origin:

    A. thyroxine.

    B. progesterone.

    C. corticotrophin (ACTH).

    D. insulin.

    E. thyrotrophin.

25. Regarding oestrogen production in pregnancy:

    A. the placenta synthesizes oestriol from pregnenolone.

    B. urinary oestriol levels reflect the pattern of plasma oestriol.

    C. the fetal liver hydroxylates DHA sulphate.

    D. the fetal adrenal is involved indirectly in oestriol production.

    E. the normal placenta has an active sulphatase system.

26. Prolactin:

    A. is secreted in response to suckling.

    B. is a polypeptide.

    C. is produced by the acidophil cells of the posterior lobe of the pituitary gland.

    D. is under inhibitory control.

    E. closely resembles thyrotrophin-releasing hormone (TRH).

27. Luteinizing hormone-releasing hormone (LHRH):

    A. is a decapeptide hormone.

    B. releases follicle-stimulating hormone (FSH) as well as LH.

    C. is stored in the posterior pituitary.

    D. is controlled by neurotransmitters.

    E. is secreted continuously.

28. During starvation:

    A. plasma free fatty acids increase.

    B. plasma insulin increases.

    C. plasma reverse tri-iodothyronine increases.

    D. plasma glucagon increases.

    E. liver glycogen falls.

29. The pancreatic islets produce the following hormones:

    A. cholecystokinin.

    B. glucagon.

    C. secretin.

    D. vasoactive intestinal polypeptide (VIP).

    E. insulin.

30. In the regulation of glucose metabolism:

    A. insulin promotes the uptake of glucose by muscle cells.

    B. glucose-6-phosphatase occurs in muscle but not in liver cells.

    C. adrenaline promotes the breakdown of hepatic glycogen.

    D. lactic acid is the end product of the aerobic metabolism of glucose.

    E. insulin is secreted by the delta cells of the islets of Langerhans.

31. Growth hormone secretion:

A. is from acidophil cells in the anterior pituitary gland.

B. is inhibited by somatostatin.

C. is increased by glucose.

D. leads to increased protein synthesis.

E. falls in response to exercise.

32. The following drugs cross the placenta:

A. aspirin.

B. warfarin.

C. heparin.

D. RU486.

E. paracetamol.

33. Oxytocin:

A. is a steroid hormone.

B. is produced in the anterior lobe of the pituitary gland.

C. is inactivated by oxytocinase.

D. has an antidiuretic effect greater than that of antidiuretic hormone.

E. may be used for induction of labour.

34. Glucose-6-phosphate:

A. is formed from glucose and adenosine triphosphate (ATP).

B. is hydrolysed by glucose-6-phosphatase to glucose and inorganic phosphate.

C. is a 'high-energy' phosphate ester.

D. is transported by the blood from the liver to all body tissues.

E. is excreted in large amounts by infants suffering from galactosaemia.

35. Glucagon:

A. is secreted by delta cells of the islets of Langerhans in the pancreas.

B. is a polypeptide containing 29 amino acids.

    C. can be used in the emergency treatment of hyperglycaemia.

    D. is released in response to exercise.

    E. acts on adipose tissue.

36. **Vasopressin:**

    A. is synthesized and stored in the posterior lobe of the pituitary gland.

    B. contains nine amino acids.

    C. is released in response to a fall in plasma osmolality.

    D. acts on the renal collecting tubules to reduce their permeability to water.

    E. is an important pressor agent.

37. **Aldosterone:**

    A. is produced by the fetal adrenal gland.

    B. causes sodium and potassium retention.

    C. is secreted by the zona glomerulosa of the adrenal cortex in response to angiotensin II.

    D. is the only adrenal hormone with mineralocorticoid properties.

    E. increases blood volume.

38. **During the climacteric:**

    A. oestrogen is the first steroid hormone to become deficient.

    B. FSH levels rise before those of LH.

    C. oestrone is the predominant oestrogen postmenopausally.

    D. testosterone is the main precursor of oestrogen postmenopausally.

    E. prolactin levels fall.

39. **Raised levels of serum FSH are found in:**

    A. association with the use of the oral contraceptive pill.

    B. postmenopausal women.

    C. association with the use of LHRH analogues.

    D. panhypopituitarism.

    E. pure gonadal dysgenesis.

40. Bromocriptine:

    A. is a derivative of ergot.

    B. causes inhibition of dopaminergic receptors at the pituitary level.

    C. causes raised prolactin levels to return to normal after 24–48 hours of starting the treatment.

    D. is teratogenic if taken during the first trimester.

    E. causes dizziness.

41. Organisms associated with infection of the female urinary tract include:

    A. *Escherichia coli.*

    B. *Mycobacterium tuberculosis.*

    C. *Staphylococcus pyogenes.*

    D. *Proteus mirabilis.*

    E. Döderlein's bacillus.

42. Normally there is no commensal flora in the:

    A. appendix.

    B. external auditory meatus.

    C. trachea.

    D. vagina.

    E. nasal vestibule.

43. Bacterial plasmids:

    A. are associated with genetic transfer by conjugation.

    B. exist as self-replicating extra-chromosomal DNA.

    C. occur only in Gram-negative species.

    D. may be transferred between different genera.

    E. may confer multiple antibiotic resistance.

44. Bacterial flagella:

    A. are the locomotive organs of bacteria.

    B. are associated with transfer of drug resistance.

    C. are characteristic of Gram-positive organisms.

    D. can bring about haemagglutination.

    E. may be responsible for bacteriophages in certain bacteria.

45. **Chlamydia differ from viruses in the following respects:**

    A. they possess both RNA and DNA.

    B. they multiply by binary fission.

    C. they have ribosomes.

    D. they have cell walls.

    E. they have metabolically active enzymes.

46. **The following organisms commonly cause acute meningitis:**

    A. *Haemophilus influenzae.*

    B. *Neisseria meningitidis.*

    C. *beta-haemolytic streptococcus.*

    D. *Staphylococcus albus.*

    E. *Diplococcus pneumonia.*

47. **Passive immunization:**

    A. is contraindicated during pregnancy.

    B. should not be used in patients with hypogammaglobulinaemia.

    C. may lead to graft-versus-host disease in patients with marrow aplasia.

    D. is the normal mode of protection against infection up to the age of 6 months.

    E. may lead to serum sickness.

48. **Immunoglobulin (Ig):**

    A. class M (IgM) is transferred across the placenta.

    B. class G (IgG) has a molecular weight of 150 000.

    C. class M (IgM) is produced in primary immune response.

    D. class E (IgE) is responsible for type I allergic reaction.

    E. class G (IgG) in the human newborn is mainly of maternal origin.

49. Neutrophils:

    A. phagocytose bacteria and fungi.

    B. predominate in acute inflammatory conditions.

    C. synthesize transcobalamin III.

    D. have a life span of 12 days.

    E. synthesize antibodies.

50. Characteristically viruses:

    A. derive energy from host cells.

    B. reproduce only within living cells.

    C. are fully organized and infectious throughout their life cycle.

    D. grow in mature human erythrocytes from susceptible individuals.

    E. have specific proteins which may inhibit host cell DNA synthesis.

51. Side-effects of bleomycin include:

    A. hypothermia.

    B. skin pigmentation.

    C. alopecia.

    D. mucositis.

    E. pulmonary fibrosis which is reduced by oxygen administration.

52. Side-effects of cyclophosphamide include:

    A. haematuria.

    B. peripheral neuropathy.

    C. alopecia.

    D. gonadal damage.

    E. nausea and vomiting.

53. Streptomycin:

    A. has more activity in alkaline urine.

    B. is water-soluble.

    C. is primarily bacteriostatic.

  D. is potentially nephrotoxic.

  E. is eliminated in its conjugated form by the kidney.

54. **Morphine:**

  A. is not absorbed after oral intake.

  B. causes release of antidiuretic hormone.

  C. is potentiated by neostigmine.

  D. depresses the vomiting centre.

  E. causes meiosis.

55. **The following drugs are contraindicated in breast-feeding mothers:**

  A. lithium carbonate.

  B. warfarin.

  C. propylthiouracil.

  D. penicillamine.

  E. insulin.

56. **The uptake of glucose by the erythrocyte:**

  A. is an example of facilitated diffusion.

  B. requires hydrolysis of ATP.

  C. is saturable.

  D. is inhibited by ouabain.

  E. is analogous to the uptake of glucose by *Escherichia coli*.

57. **Histamine:**

  A. causes release of adrenaline from the suprarenal medulla.

  B. causes local vasoconstriction in the skin.

  C. increases gastric acid secretion.

  D. can cause throbbing headache.

  E. is found in mast cell granules.

58. **Heparin:**

  A. is a mucopolysaccharide.

  B. can lead to thrombocytopaenia.

   C. crosses the placenta.

   D. is contraindicated in breast-feeding mothers.

   E. can lead to bone demineralization.

59. Ethyl alcohol:

   A. acts as a diuretic by inhibiting the secretion of antidiuretic hormone (ADH).

   B. is a central nervous system (CNS) stimulant.

   C. has no calorific value.

   D. excessive intake during pregnancy can lead to fetal intr auterine growth retardation.

   E. enhances the action of sedatives and hypnotics.

60. Congenital abnormalities may be caused by antenatal maternal ingestion of:

   A. warfarin.

   B. phenytoin.

   C. ampicillin.

   D. ethambutol.

   E. ethionamide.

Paper 2 (Questions 61–120):

61. The increase in cardiac output in pregnancy:

   A. occurs mainly in the first 20 weeks.

   B. results from an increased stroke volume.

   C. results from an increased pulse rate.

   D. decreases in the last trimester.

   E. is more in physically fit mothers than in those who do not regularly exercise.

62. In a creatinine clearance test where: plasma concentration = 3.5 mg/dl, urine concentration = 0.504 g/L and urine volume = 2 L/24 hours, the following statements are correct:

   A. total amount of creatinine secreted per day = 1800 mg.

   B. total amount of creatinine secreted per minute = 0.7 mg.

   C. creatinine clearance = 20 ml/min.

   D. if the patient was pregnant she would have normal renal function.

   E. the concentration of creatinine in the renal vein would be 3.7 mg/dl.

63. **In a patient with the following results: pH = 7.0, PCO_2 = 80 mmHg, standard bicarbonate = 25 mEq/L:**

   A. it is likely that she has a metabolic acidosis.

   B. the hydrogen ion concentration would be 0.00009 mmol/L.

   C. the patient would be cyanosed.

   D. the patient could have chronic bronchitis.

   E. the patient could have fibrosing alveolitis.

64. **During normal pregnancy:**

   A. plasma volume increases by about 40%.

   B. erythrocyte sedimentation rate (ESR) rises.

   C. iron binding capacity falls.

   D. venous blood pressure falls.

   E. packed cell volume falls.

65. **Ventilation:**

   A. is increased in hypoxia due to stimulation of the central chemoreceptors.

   B. is increased in respiratory acidosis.

   C. is decreased by the administration of veratrum alkaloid.

   D. is increased in hyperthermia due to stimulation of the peripheral chemoreceptors.

   E. is stimulated by J receptors in the airways.

66. **Angiotensin II:**

   A. is a decapeptide.

   B. leads to aldosterone secretion.

   C. concentration rises in the infant from birth to age 1 year.

    D. is a vasoconstrictor agent.

    E. is converted into angiotensin I in the lungs.

67. **2,3-Diphosphoglycerate (2,3-DPG):**

    A. shifts the oxygen dissociation curve to the left.

    B. is increased by androgens.

    C. has lower levels in fetal red cells than in adult cells.

    D. is produced in the Krebs cycle (indirect glycolysis).

    E. levels rise during the first week of life.

68. **Normal urodynamic findings in the adult female include:**

    A. voiding pressure = 45–70 mmHg.

    B. maximum urine flow rate = 20–40 ml/s.

    C. maximum urethral pressure in the absence of micturition = 50-100 cm H_2O.

    D. voiding volume = 200–350 ml.

    E. bladder capacity = 600–750 ml.

69. **Colostrum:**

    A. contains antibodies to *E. coli.*

    B. has more protein and fat than mature human milk.

    C. has less carbohydrate than cow milk.

    D. contains epidermal growth factors.

    E. contains steroid hormones.

70. **Substances essential to the development of the red blood cells include:**

    A. folinic acid.

    B. ascorbic acid.

    C. nicotinic acid.

    D. methotrexate.

    E. cyanocobalamine.

71. **Iron metabolism in normal adults:**

    A. iron is absorbed in the ferric form.

    B. the fetus gets its iron from the mother by passive transport across the placenta.

C. the earliest effect of iron deficiency anaemia on the erythrocyte is a reduction in the mean corpuscular volume (MCV).

D. iron deficiency anaemia is a macrocytic anaemia.

E. iron stores are assessed by measuring serum iron levels.

72. **The increase in uterine blood flow in pregnancy is contributed to by:**

A. increased number of uterine arterioles.

B. increased diameter of placental bed vessels.

C. reduced arterio-venous resistance in the placenta.

D. reduced angiotensin II levels.

E. increased blood volume.

73. **Changes in liver function in normal pregnancy include:**

A. an increase in the heat-stable fraction of serum alkaline phosphatase.

B. a rise in aspartate aminotransferase.

C. a rise in serum albumin.

D. a rise in serum cholesterol.

E. a fall in total protein concentration.

74. **Changes in respiratory function in normal pregnancy include:**

A. an increase in respiratory rate.

B. an increase in vital capacity.

C. a reduction in residual volume.

D. an increase in oxygen consumption.

E. an increase in minute volume.

75. **The heart rate:**

A. is increased in pregnancy.

B. is increased in hypothermia.

C. is increased with ritodrine.

D. is normally a reflection of the activity of the sino-atrial node.

E. may be decreased in obstructive jaundice.

76. Disseminated intravascular coagulation:

   A. occurs as a primary phenomenon.

   B. is associated with missed abortion.

   C. may affect myometrial function.

   D. may not be associated with haemorrhage.

   E. can be diagnosed by finding fibrinogen degradation products in plasma.

77. Fetal haemoglobin (Hb F):

   A. has a high oxygen affinity.

   B. contains alpha and beta chains.

   C. shifts the oxygen dissociation curve to the left.

   D. is the only type of haemoglobin present during the intrauterine life.

   E. is resistant to denaturation by strong alkali.

78. In the normal adult human:

   A. the PR interval should not exceed 0.3.

   B. the second heart sound represents aortic and mitral valves closure.

   C. ejection from the left ventricle occurs during the period of isometric contraction phase.

   D. contraction of the atria contributes about one-third of ventricular filling.

   E. ventricular systole precedes ventricular depolarization.

79. Respiratory acidosis may be caused by:

   A. pH fall due to renal failure.

   B. voluntary hyperventilation.

   C. uretero-sigmoid anastomosis.

   D. chronic bronchitis.

   E. excessive sedation.

80. Vasoconstriction in the systemic circulation:

   A. can occur due to chemoreceptor stimulation.

   B. is mediated by the vagus nerve when there is hypotension.

    C. is caused by local accumulation of lactate.

    D. causes a rise in peripheral resistance.

    E. may be caused by the administration of syntometrine.

81. Increased vascular permeability in acute inflammation may be due to:

    A. histamine.

    B. serotonin.

    C. cortisol.

    D. plasma kinins.

    E. globulin permeability factor.

82. The following statements regarding cellular damage are correct:

    A. in hyaline degeneration the cytoplasm is eosinophilic.

    B. hydropic degeneration is irreversible.

    C. pyknosis refers to nuclear shrinkage and clumping of chromatin.

    D. striated muscles may undergo necrosis in acute fevers.

    E. karyorrhexis refers to nuclear digestion.

83. Hormone secreting tumours of the ovary include:

    A. granulosa cell tumour.

    B. Brenner tumour.

    C. arrhenoblastoma.

    D. dysgerminoma.

    E. fibroma.

84. The following are histological features of sarcoidosis:

    A. Schaumann bodies.

    B. Langhan giant cells.

    C. round cell infiltration.

    D. caseation.

    E. epitheloid cells.

85. Cancer ovary:

    A. has an overall 5-year survival rate of 75%.

    B. the omentum is a frequent site for metastases.

    C. pelvic irradiation is a predisposing factor.

    D. histologically is most commonly of germ cell origin.

    E. is more common in women with positive family history.

86. Regarding the effect of ionizing radiation on tissue:

    A. epithelial cells are more sensitive than connective tissue cells.

    B. bones and muscles are relatively radioresistant.

    C. can lead to delayed meiosis.

    D. high local oxygen concentration is protective.

    E. may cause osteosarcoma.

87. The following conditions are inherited as X-linked recessive:

    A. galactosaemia.

    B. cystic fibrosis.

    C. haemophilia.

    D. Christmas disease.

    E. nephrogenic diabetes insipidus.

88. Phagocytosis is a function of:

    A. neutrophils.

    B. lymphocytes.

    C. histiocytes.

    D. squamous cells.

    E. eosinophil polymorphonuclear leucocytes.

89. Mitochondria:

    A. are found in all prokaryotic cells.

    B. are found in all eukaryotic cells.

    C. contain DNA.

    D. contain ribosomes.

    E. store energy as ATP.

90. The following are endodermal in origin:

A. the heart.

B. the spleen.

C. the adrenal cortex.

D. the dermis.

E. the germ cells.

91. The following are tumours which characteristically arise in the ovary:

A. melanoma.

B. seminoma.

C. teratoma.

D. endometrioid carcinoma.

E. endodermal sinus tumour.

92. An embolus can be formed of:

A. tumour cells.

B. trophoblastic cells.

C. gas.

D. amniotic fluid.

E. silica particles.

93. In the normal adult human heart:

A. the sino-atrial node is located in the wall of the right atrium.

B. the atrio-ventricular node is located in the superior wall of the right ventricle.

C. there is a delay in the conduction of the cardiac impulse at the atrio-ventricular node.

D. the second heart sound is caused by the closure of the aortic and pulmonary valves.

E. there is no blood flow from the left atrium into the left ventricle during diastole.

94. Platelets:

A. have similar counts in adults and normal term infants.

B. have an intravascular life span of 21–28 days.

    C. are derived from megakaryocytes.

    D. play a significant role in the prevention of haemorrhage from the placental bed at the end of the third stage of labour.

    E. are increased in number postpartum.

95. **The following tumours are of embryonic origin:**

    A. dermoid cyst.

    B. nephroblastoma.

    C. glioblastoma.

    D. reticulum cell sarcoma.

    E. retinoblastoma.

96. **Regarding human cell structure:**

    A. ribosomes contain RNA and DNA.

    B. histones are very acidic proteins which bind DNA and are involved in producing higher-order structures of chromatin.

    C. nucleolus organizer regions exist on chromosomes 13, 14, 15, 21 and 22.

    D. nuclear RNA is a precursor of cytoplasmic ribosomal RNA.

    E. each chromosome contains a single separate DNA molecule.

97. **Histones:**

    A. are the major proteins present in chromatin.

    B. are basic proteins.

    C. are coded in the DNA in multiple copies.

    D. constitute the nuclear receptors for steroid hormones.

    E. are rich in lysine and arginine.

98. **The major chemical constituents of gallstones are:**

    A. cholesterol.

    B. calcium salts.

    C. uric acid.

    D. bilirubin.

    E. magnesium salts.

99. The first maturation division of the primary oocyte results in:

    A. haploid number of chromosomes.

    B. two cells of equal size.

    C. secondary oocyte and first polar body.

    D. the formation of oogonia.

    E. introduction of new DNA molecules in the cell.

100. Normal seminal fluid analysis:

    A. volume of 2–5 ml.

    B. acidic pH.

    C. does not form a coagulum.

    D. count = 20 million sperm/ml.

    E. motility = 40%.

101. The following are essential amino acids:

    A. lysine.

    B. valine.

    C. phenylalanine.

    D. leucine.

    E. tyrosine.

102. Beta-oxidation of long-chain fatty acids:

    A. occurs in the mitochondrial matrix of the cell.

    B. means that the fatty acid is broken down by removing two carbon atoms at a time.

    C. yields products which can be used to synthesize glucose.

    D. is a preferential energy source during periods of rapid exercise.

    E. produces NADH and $FADH_2$ as sources of ATP production.

103. Glucose transport into the muscle is:

    A. active.

    B. inhibited by cellular energy.

    C. rate-limiting to glucose metabolism.

    D. a symport system.

    E. dependent on extracellular sodium.

104. Placental transfer of amino acids:

    A. occurs even when fetal blood levels are higher than maternal.

    B. is a mediated diffusion process.

    C. is not inhibited by anoxia.

    D. is a blood flow-limited process.

    E. is necessary for fetal growth.

105. The urea cycle:

    A. supplies the daily requirement for arginine in the newborn.

    B. converts urea to uric acid.

    C. converts ammonia to urea.

    D. acts as an energy-supplying mechanism.

    E. converts urea to ammonia and carbon dioxide.

106. In carbohydrate metabolism:

    A. glycolysis is the main aerobic metabolic pathway.

    B. excessive carbohydrate intake increases body weight due to increased carbohydrate stores.

    C. complete breakdown of a glucose molecule under normal conditions yields 38 ATP molecules.

    D. adrenaline mobilizes liver and muscle glycogen.

    E. intravenous glucose results in a greater release of insulin than oral intake.

107. Vitamin A (retinol):

    A. is fat-soluble.

    B. has limited reserves in the liver.

    C. may be teratogenic in high doses.

    D. is exclusively from plant sources.

    E. is important for night vision.

108. Regarding diagnostic ultrasound scan:

    A. the resolution is directly proportional to the frequency used.

    B. the focal length is directly proportional to the frequency used.

    C. the resolution along the direction of the beam is finer than that across its width.

    D. frequencies used are in the range 1–10 MHz.

    E. bowel gas enables clearer imaging of underlying structures.

109. Regarding ionizing radiations:

    A. beta particles are negatively charged electrons.

    B. gamma rays are generated by the circulating electrons of the atom.

    C. megavoltage gamma rays have a more skin-damaging effect than conventional X-ray.

    D. 1 Gray is equal to 1 Joule per kg.

    E. can lead to abnormal mitosis.

110. The plasma levels of the following hormones are increased during normal pregnancy:

    A. ACTH.

    B. aldosterone.

    C. cortisol.

    D. prolactin.

    E. TSH.

111. The following are actively transferred across the human placenta:

    A. glucose.

    B. alanine.

    C. potassium.

    D. calcium.

    E. vitamin A.

112. In fat metabolism:

    A. digestion and absorption of fat are impaired in the absence of pancreatic enzymes.

    B. linoleic and linolenic acids are essential unsaturated fatty acids.

    C. 1 g yields 9 kcal.

    D. lipaemia represents an abnormal state of fat absorption.

    E. glucose concentration in the blood controls fat metabolism.

113. The following separate maternal and fetal blood in the human placenta:

    A. trophoblast.

    B. maternal vascular endothelium.

    C. fetal vascular endothelium.

    D. maternal connective tissue.

    E. fetal connective tissue.

114. In the normal fetus and newborn:

    A. prostaglandins enhance closure of the ductus arteriosus after birth.

    B. there is an increase in the renal blood flow after delivery.

    C. the CNS is fully mature at birth.

    D. the ductus venosus conveys oxygenated blood before birth.

    E. there is high pulmonary vascular resistance before birth.

115. During normal fetal development:

    A. the first pharyngeal pouch forms the Eustacian tube.

    B. the artery of the fifth pharyngeal arch forms the pulmonary artery.

    C. the second pharyngeal pouch forms the superior parathyroid glands.

    D. the artery of the third pharyngeal arch forms part of the internal carotid artery.

    E. the first pharyngeal arch forms the laryngeal cartilages.

116. In multiple pregnancy:

- **A.** the number of chorionic sacs is always equal to the number of ova fertilized.
- **B.** conjoined twins result from splitting of the germinal disc after the appearance of the primitive streak.
- **C.** a diamniotic placenta is only found in dizygotic twins.
- **D.** the placentas of dizygotic twins may become fused macroscopically.
- **E.** there is high maternal serum alpha-feto protein.

117. Regarding fetal physiology:

- **A.** the pH of fetal blood rises throughout the normal first stage of labour.
- **B.** there is a high pulmonary vascular resistance.
- **C.** the heart starts beating at 22 days after fertilization.
- **D.** the pH of the fetal blood is independent of the maternal blood pH.
- **E.** fetal breathing movements are usually increased in labour.

118. The following statements regarding the term fetus are correct:

- **A.** the suboccipito-bregmatic diameter is 13 cm.
- **B.** the submento-bregmatic diameter is 9.5 cm.
- **C.** the mento-vertical diameter is 13 cm.
- **D.** the occipito-frontal diameter is the presenting diameter in brow presentation.
- **E.** the bitrochanteric diameter is 9 cm.

119. In the fetus:

- **A.** the coronal suture lies between the two parietal bones.
- **B.** the umbilical cord normally contains one artery and two veins.
- **C.** the placental-fetal weight ratio at full term is of the order of 1:6.
- **D.** entanglement of the umbilical cords is common in twin pregnancy.
- **E.** the anterior fontanelle is easily felt on vaginal examination when the head is fully flexed.

120. The following are homologous organs in the male and female respectively:

  A. prostate and Skene's duct.

  B. scrotum and labium minor.

  C. Cowper's gland and Bartholin's gland.

  D. corpus spongiosum and vestibular bulb.

  E. gubernaculum of testis and round ligament of ovary.

Paper 3 (Questions 121–180):

121. The cervix:

  A. undergoes cyclical changes during the menstrual cycle.

  B. sheds its lining at menstruation.

  C. has a lining of columnar epithelium which changes abruptly into stratified squamous epithelium at the squamo-columnar junction.

  D. has a large number of glands opening on to its vaginal surface.

  E. has a peritoneal covering on the posterior surface of its supravaginal part.

122. The trigon of the bladder:

  A. is the least sensitive part of the bladder.

  B. is derived from endoderm.

  C. is the least distensible part of the bladder.

  D. is darker than the rest of the bladder.

  E. lies between the internal urethral orifice and the ureteric orifices.

123. The inguinal ligament:

  A. is attached to the anterior and posterior superior iliac spines.

  B. is part of the internal oblique muscle.

  C. has the lacunar ligament attached to its medial end.

  D. has the ilio-inguinal nerve inferior to it.

  E. has the femoral sheath deep to it.

124. The superficial perineal pouch in the female:

   A. contains the bulb of the vestibule.

   B. contains branches of the internal pudendal artery.

   C. contains the ischiocavernosus muscles.

   D. contains the external sphincter of the urethra.

   E. lies between the two layers of the urogenital diaphragm.

125. The anal canal:

   A. is lined entirely by mucous columnar epithelium.

   B. is developed entirely from the hind gut.

   C. has a blood supply from the internal pudendal artery.

   D. has a sphincter consisting of smooth muscles.

   E. has lymph vessels which drain to the superficial inguinal lymph nodes.

126. The broad ligament:

   A. has the ovary attached to its posterior surface.

   B. has the Fallopian tube in its upper free border.

   C. has the ovarian artery in its lower attached border.

   D. has the round ligament forming a ridge on its posterior surface.

   E. has the ureter passing forwards in its lower attached border.

127. Fetal haemoglobin (Hb F):

   A. appears in the fetal circulation at 20 weeks gestation.

   B. is found in adult patients with thalassaemia.

   C. is not detected in healthy adults.

   D. comprises about 90% of the haemoglobin in the term newborn.

   E. is detected by the Kleihauer test.

128. Germ cells:

   A. arise in the primitive gut mesentery of the embryo.

   B. multiply by mitotic division.

   C. enter prophase of meiosis I only after puberty in the testis.

    D.   replicate the amount of chromosomal DNA at the beginning of mitosis and meiosis.

    E.   show marked degeneration in the latter half of fetal life in the gonads of both sexes.

129. Structures arising from Wolffian remnants include:

    A.   the epoöphoron.

    B.   the processus vaginalis.

    C.   the paraoöphoron.

    D.   the round ligament.

    E.   Gaertner's duct.

130. During meiosis:

    A.   there are two replications with one cell division.

    B.   bivalents are seen during 1st prophase.

    C.   the two components of the bivalent are attached by their centromere.

    D.   chiasmata become visible during 1st prophase.

    E.   one member of each pair of chromosomes moves to the opposite poles of the cell during 1st anaphase.

131. The anterior pituitary gland produces:

    A.   oxytocin.

    B.   vasopressin.

    C.   growth hormone.

    D.   gonadotrophin-releasing hormone.

    E.   prolactin.

132. Free (unbound) thyroxine in plasma:

    A.   is less than 1% of total thyroxine levels.

    B.   regulates TSH secretion.

    C.   is free to enter cells and bind to nuclear receptors.

    D.   is raised in myxoedema.

    E.   is raised in pregnancy.

133. In the control of pituitary-adrenal function:
   A. the stress response overrides the diurnal rhythm.
   B. cortisol levels are normally maximal at 08:00 hour.
   C. there is negative feedback from 17-hydroxyprogesterone.
   D. cortisol binding globulin plays a part.
   E. corticotrophin-releasing factor is a glycoprotein.

134. Human chorionic gonadotrophin (hCG):
   A. is a glycoprotein.
   B. has a sub-unit similar to FSH.
   C. reaches a peak level at about 20 weeks gestation.
   D. is thought to stimulate fetal testosterone secretion.
   E. is produced by syncytiotrophoblast.

135. Oxytocin is:
   A. a lipid hormone.
   B. synthesized in hypothalamic nuclei.
   C. secreted directly from its site of production.
   D. secreted in short bursts in the second stage of labour.
   E. important in the production of uterine contractions in early pregnancy.

136. Adrenal androgens:
   A. are important precursors of oestrogen in postmenopausal women.
   B. are synthesized from cortisol.
   C. secretion is controlled by ACTH.
   D. are important in the onset of puberty.
   E. are secreted by the zona glomerulosa.

137. Regarding immunoglobulin (Ig) in the human fetus and neonate:
   A. maternal IgA is placentally transferred from 32–40 weeks gestation.
   B. IgM is the first Ig to be synthesized in the fetus.

    C. transfer of maternal IgG across the placenta is an active process.

    D. all maternal IgG has been catabolized in a normal infant by 3 weeks of life.

    E. breast milk IgA is absorbed by the infant's small intestine for up to 6 months of life.

138. Bacterial capsules:

    A. act as virulence factors.

    B. may be demonstrated by either positive or negative staining.

    C. are all composed of polysaccharide.

    D. swell with specific antisera.

    E. formation is promoted by serial culture *in vitro*.

139. Hypersensitivity reactions include:

    A. arthus reaction.

    B. contact dermatitis.

    C. Shick's test.

    D. tuberculin reaction.

    E. Ptyriasis versicolor.

140. Organisms that have an important natural reservoir other than man include:

    A. *Bordetella pertussis.*

    B. *Listeria monocytogenes.*

    C. *Vibrio para-haemolyticus.*

    D. *Neisseria gonorrhoeae.*

    E. *Treponema pallidum.*

141. During pregnancy:

    A. the half-life of antibiotics excreted by the kidney may increase.

    B. glomerular filtration rate decreases.

    C. orally administered drugs may be more slowly absorbed.

    D. anti-malaria prophylaxis should not be given.

    E. oral ketocanazole is contraindicated.

142. The incubation period of:

    A. rubella is 14–21 days.

    B. gonorrhoea is 2–5 days.

    C. chickenpox is 14–21 days.

    D. malaria is 10–14 days.

    E. whooping cough is 7–10 days.

143. Human immune-deficiency virus (HIV):

    A. is a member of the herpes group of viruses.

    B. could be transmitted transplacentally.

    C. is inactivated by heating at 56°C for 30 minutes.

    D. is inactivated by nonoxynol-9.

    E. causes hypergammaglobulinaemia.

144. Congenital infection or abnormality could be caused by:

    A. *Treponema pallidum.*

    B. *Toxoplasma gondii.*

    C. *Plasmodium falciparum.*

    D. Cytomegalovirus.

    E. *Salmonella typhi.*

145. Erythromycin:

    A. is a beta-lactam antibiotic.

    B. crosses the placenta to achieve a concentration comparable to the maternal serum concentration.

    C. is used as a substitute for penicillin in allergic patients.

    D. is a suitable treatment for Legionnaire's disease.

    E. is active against *Mycoplasma hominis.*

146. Organisms commonly sensitive to penicillin include:

    A. *Treponema pallidum.*

    B. Beta-haemolytic streptococcus.

    C. *Chlamydia trachomatis.*

    D. *Staphylococcus aureus.*

    E. *Neisseria meningitidis.*

147. Recognized side-effects of prostaglandins include:

    A. high temperature.

    B. vomiting.

    C. diarrhoea.

    D. bronchodilatation.

    E. uterine rupture.

148. Recognized side-effects of beta-sympathomymetics include:

    A. hyperglycaemia.

    B. hyperkalaemia.

    C. tachycardia.

    D. hypertension.

    E. pulmonary oedema.

149. Progesterone:

    A. stimulates the synthesis of oestrogen receptors.

    B. stimulates the epithelial cells of the Fallopian tubes to secrete mucus.

    C. is thermogenic.

    D. is synthesized in the adrenal medulla.

    E. is used in the treatment of endometrial carcinoma.

150. Regarding cytotoxic drugs:

    A. nitrogen mustard drugs are antimetabolites.

    B. cyclophosphamide is an alkylating agent.

    C. methotrexate is an antimetabolite.

    D. androgens have beneficial effects in some cases of breast cancer.

    E. cisplatin is a vinca alkaloid.

151. In pregnancy:

    A. oxygen consumption increases by 50 ml/min.

    B. PCO_2 falls compared to the non-pregnant state.

C. the ratio of FEV1/FVC is increased.

D. residual volume is decreased.

E. there is increased sensitivity of the respiratory centres to CO_2.

152. **In a patient with metabolic acidosis:**

A. hypoventilation may be a cause.

B. chronic renal failure may be a cause.

C. the pH is usually greater than 7.4.

D. aspiration of vomit may be a cause.

E. hyperventilation may occur.

153. **A shift of the oxy-haemoglobin dissociation curve:**

A. to the left increases the affinity of haemoglobin to oxygen.

B. to the left increases the quantity of oxygen in combination with haemoglobin at P_{50}.

C. to the right occurs with acidosis.

D. to the left occurs with increased concentration of 2,3-DPG.

E. to the right occurs in the fetus.

154. **Regarding haemopoiesis in pregnancy:**

A. there is a parallel increase in maternal plasma volume and red cell mass.

B. maternal iron deficiency will lead to fetal iron deficiency.

C. the normal daily requirement of folic acid is 300 micrograms.

D. parenteral iron will lead to a quicker response than oral iron in cases of iron deficiency anaemia.

E. phytates reduce iron absorption from the intestines.

155. **Tocolytic agents include:**

A. ritodrine.

B. indomethacin.

C. nifedipine.

D. prostaglandin E_2.

E. oxytocin.

156. The following statements are correct:
- **A.** the lining cells of the Fallopian tube are non-ciliated.
- **B.** fertilization takes place in the Fallopian tube.
- **C.** decidual cells could be found lining the Fallopian tube during pregnancy.
- **D.** normally the lateral part of the Fallopian tube is in close contact with the ovary.
- **E.** the peritoneal covering is continuous around the Fallopian tube.

157. The following diseases are commonly made worse by pregnancy:
- **A.** rheumatoid arthritis.
- **B.** gout.
- **C.** migraine.
- **D.** pulmonary hypertension.
- **E.** bronchial asthma.

158. The following statements are correct:
- **A.** serum fibrinogen levels increase in normal pregnancy.
- **B.** prostacyclin promotes platelet aggregation.
- **C.** thromboxane causes vasodilatation.
- **D.** pre-eclampsia may be associated with thrombocytopaenia.
- **E.** venography is contraindicated in pregnancy.

159. ESR is characteristically low or normal in:
- **A.** pregnancy.
- **B.** multiple myelomatosis.
- **C.** macroglobulinaemia.
- **D.** rheumatic fever.
- **E.** defibrinated blood.

160. Ovulation occurs:
- **A.** before the biphasic rise in temperature.
- **B.** before the LH surge.

C. following follicular stimulation by FSH.

D. in some cases of amenorrhoea.

E. after disappearance of cervical mucus ferning.

161. Electroencephalogram (EEG) changes during sleep:

A. are associated with reduced skeletal muscle tone in REM sleep.

B. have the highest frequency in stage 4 of NREM sleep.

C. have alpha-like waves in NREM sleep.

D. have rapid, low voltage waves during dreaming.

E. are significantly altered in pregnancy.

162. The following conditions have a multifactorial pattern of inheritance:

A. neural tube defect.

B. cystic fibrosis.

C. Peutz's syndrome.

D. tuberose sclerosis.

E. cleft palate.

163. Testicular differentiation:

A. is associated with 46XY karyotype.

B. is never found in 47XXY patients.

C. is seen in H-Y antigen negative patients.

D. occurs before external masculinization of the fetus.

E. does not occur in Down's syndrome.

164. A 46XY individual with a female phenotype:

A. may have streak gonads.

B. can complete the biosynthesis of testosterone.

C. has a raised risk of gonadal malignancy.

D. may be unable to utilize testosterone.

E. results from oestrogen therapy given during pregnancy.

165. Pancreatitis in pregnancy is associated with:

A. alcoholism.

B. pre-eclampsia.

    C. ampicillin.

    D. thiazide diuretics.

    E. occurrence in the first trimester.

166. **The following structures are related to the antero-lateral part of the left kidney:**

    A. stomach.

    B. spleen.

    C. duodenum.

    D. jejunum.

    E. splenic vein.

167. **The following hormones promote maturation of the breast:**

    A. growth hormone.

    B. parathyroid hormone.

    C. thyroid hormone.

    D. insulin.

    E. cortisol.

168. **The following statements regarding the breast are correct:**

    A. it is mesodermal in origin.

    B. it lies within the deep fascia of the chest wall.

    C. it is an apocrine gland.

    D. thelarche occurs usually between 9 and 12 years of age.

    E. the alveoli have a rich nerve supply.

169. **Recognized causes for low plasma zinc in adults include:**

    A. diabetes mellitus.

    B. anorexia nervosa.

    C. polycystic ovarian disease.

    D. burns.

    E. nephrotic syndrome.

170. **The following are live attenuated vaccines:**

    A. pertussis vaccine.

    B. mumps vaccine.

C. rabies vaccine.

D. hepatitis B vaccine.

E. bacille Calmette-Guérin (BCG).

171. Causes of hypokalaemia include:

A. vomiting.

B. insulin deficiency.

C. beta-adrenergic blocking drugs.

D. aldosteronism.

E. catabolic states.

172. The following changes occur in normal pregnancy:

A. the central venous pressure increases.

B. the systemic vascular resistance decreases.

C. the pulmonary vascular resistance increases.

D. the pulmonary arterial pressure increases.

E. the renal blood flow increases.

173. Drugs which stimulate alpha-adrenergic receptors include:

A. phenoxybenzamine.

B. phentolamine.

C. metaraminol.

D. methoxamine.

E. phenylephrine.

174. The following drugs augment the anticoagulant effect of warfarin:

A. cimetidine.

B. ketocanazole.

C. phenytoin.

D. rifampicin.

E. metronidazole.

175. The following drugs are alkylating agents:

A. methotrexate.

B. melphalan.

    C. chlorambucil.

    D. cyclophosphamide.

    E. nitrogen mustard.

176. The following increase the risk of having a baby with neural tube defect:

    A. folic acid.

    B. sodium valproate.

    C. family history.

    D. increased maternal age.

    E. heparin.

177. The efficiency of placental transfer increases in the third trimester because:

    A. placental growth becomes faster than fetal growth.

    B. vasculo-syncytial membranes develop.

    C. the surface area available for transport increases.

    D. maternal and fetal blood flows become countercurrent.

    E. the syncytiotrophoblast gets thinner.

178. The following antirheumatic drugs are not contraindicated in breast-feeding mothers:

    A. naproxen.

    B. diclofenac.

    C. mefenamic acid.

    D. flurbiprofen.

    E. ibuprofen.

179. Regarding the use of Doppler ultrasound in obstetrics:

    A. the Doppler-shifted signals from blood vessels are within the audible range.

    B. the normal umbilical artery has a high-resistance flow pattern.

    C. the frequencies used are 20–100 MHz.

    D. the pulsatility index is independent of the angle of insonation.

    E. the diastolic frequencies are directly proportional to the peripheral resistance.

180. **In nuclear magnetic resonance imaging:**

    A. relaxation constants are measured in two planes.

    B. one Tesla equals 10 000 G.

    C. fetal movement during imaging enhances resolution.

    D. fatty tissue produces high intensity signals.

    E. the technique is not contraindicated in pregnancy.

▌ MCQ ANSWERS

The true answers are given below:

Paper 1			
1. ADE	**29.** BDE	**58.** ABE	**85.** BCE
2. ADE	**30.** AC	**59.** ADE	**86.** ABCE
3. ABD	**31.** ABD	**60.** ABE	**87.** CDE
4. BCDE	**32.** ABDE		**88.** ACE
5. D	**33.** CE	**Paper 2**	**89.** CDE
6. DE	**34.** AB	**61.** ABC	**90.** E
7. ABCE	**35.** BDE	**62.** BC	**91.** CDE
8. AD	**36.** B	**63.** D	**92.** ABCD
9. ABE	**37.** CE	**64.** ABE	**93.** ACD
10. ABC	**38.** BCE	**65.** BCDE	**94.** ACE
11. ABDE	**39.** BE	**66.** BD	**95.** ABE
12. CD	**40.** AE	**67.** BCDE	**96.** CDE
13. ABE	**41.** ABCD	**68.** BCDE	**97.** ABCE
14. ABCD	**42.** C	**69.** ACDE	**98.** ABD
15. BCD	**43.** ABDE	**70.** ABE	**99.** AC
16. ABCE	**44.** BD	**71.** C	**100.** ADE
17. ACD	**45.** ABCDE	**72.** BCE	**101.** ABCD
18. ABE	**46.** ABE	**73.** ADE	**102.** ABE
19. ACD	**47.** E	**74.** CDE	**103.** BC
20. BD	**48.** BCDE	**75.** ACDE	**104.** AE
21. ABD	**49.** ABC	**76.** BCD	**105.** C
22. ACD	**50.** ABE	**77.** CE	**106.** CD
23. ADE	**51.** BCD	**78.** AD	**107.** ACE
24. B	**52.** ACDE	**79.** DE	**108.** ACD
25. BCDE	**53.** ABD	**80.** ADE	**109.** ADE
26. ABD	**54.** BCE	**81.** ABDE	**110.** BCD
27. ABD	**55.** AD	**82.** ACD	**111.** BD
28. ACDE	**56.** AC	**83.** ACD	**112.** ABCE
	57. ACDE	**84.** ABE	**113.** ACE

114. BDE	**130.** BDE	**148.** ACE	**166.** ABDE
115. AD	**131.** CE	**149.** BCE	**167.** ABCDE
116. BDE	**132.** ABC	**150.** BCD	**168.** CD
117. BC	**133.** AB	**151.** ABDE	**169.** ABDE
118. BCE	**134.** ABDE	**152.** BE	**170.** BE
119. C	**135.** BD	**153.** AC	**171.** AD
120. ACDE	**136.** ACD	**154.** CE	**172.** BDE
	137. BC	**155.** ABC	**173.** CDE
Paper 3	**138.** ABD	**156.** BCD	**174.** ABE
121. ACE	**139.** ABD	**157.** D	**175.** BCDE
122. CE	**140.** BC	**158.** AD	**176.** BC
123. CE	**141.** CE	**159.** E	**177.** BCE
124. ABC	**142.** ABCDE	**160.** ACD	**178.** BCDE
125. CDE	**143.** BCDE	**161.** ACD	**179.** AD
126. ABE	**144.** ABCD	**162.** AD	**180.** ABDE
127. ABDE	**145.** CD	**163.** AD	
128. BCD	**146.** ABE	**164.** ABCD	
129. ACE	**147.** ABCE	**165.** ABCD	

15

After the Part 1: What's Next?

▌ Introduction

After you have passed the MRCOG Part 1 exam, you are usually on top of the world for a couple of weeks, basking in the glory of your success. Then, as you start to come back down to earth, you ask yourself: what's next? What was the aim of doing the Part 1 exam? Well, the only aim is to be allowed to do the Part 2 exam so you would become a Member of the Royal College of Obstetricians and Gynaecologists. Therefore, it is very appropriate to have a brief chapter about the Part 2 MRCOG preparation in the Part 1 Success Manual.

▌ Eligibility

To be allowed to sit the Part 2 exam, you have to have passed the Part 1 (hopefully in the bag by now) or have received exemption from it; worked for 4 years in a recognized post; and attended at least 8 sessions of family planning.

▌ The Part 2 Exam

The Part 2 Examination consists of a written part and an oral-assessment part. Candidates must obtain a pass mark in the written part in order to be allowed to sit the oral-assessment part. On average, 1 in 4 candidates who sit the written will pass it and be allowed to sit the oral-assessment. Of those, 3 in 4 will pass the oral-assessment and be awarded the MRCOG. This gives an overall pass rate of 1 in 5 (about 20%). Therefore the commonest cause of failure in the MRCOG Part 2 examination is failure in the written.

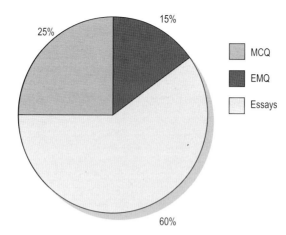

Figure 2 Contributions of the various components of the written exam to the final mark

Components of the Written Exam (see Figure 2)

1. MCQ paper: 225 questions in 1 hour and 30 minutes.
2. Short-answer essay question paper (obstetrics): 4 questions in 1 hour and 45 minutes.
3. EMQ (extended matching questions) paper: 40 questions in 1 hour.
4. Short-answer essay question paper (gynaecology): 4 questions in 1 hour and 45 minutes.

Preparing for the Part 2 exam

As you can see from the above information, the most difficult component of the Part 2 exam is the written, of which the essays form the biggest part. It is therefore necessary to start preparing for the written exam, and particularly the essays, as early as possible after passing the Part 1. Many resources are available. They include the *MRCOG Part 2 Success Manual*, a detailed book discussing exam regulations, system and format, and which provides example questions and answers in essays, MCQ, EMQ and oral assessment. There is also the *MRCOG Survival Correspondence Course* (on *http://www.mrcogcourses.co.uk*), which is particularly useful for candidates who cannot find a local trainer who is willing to correct their essays. This course can be done from anywhere in the world via e-mail or post. It provides one-to-one training and supervised practice in essays, the new EMQ and MCQ. It also contains explanatory answers and web-based resources for recent papers, hot topics, guidelines, etc. Another useful source is the *MRCOG Blog* (on *http://web.mac.com/k.sharif*). There are also many courses (for example *http://www.mrcogcourses.co.uk*) that are held regularly both in the UK and overseas (e.g. Dubai, India).